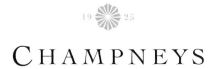

CHAMPNEYS

the cook book

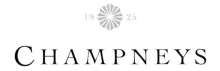

CHAMPNEYS

the cook book

—

FOOD
FOR
WELLNESS

ASTER*

to

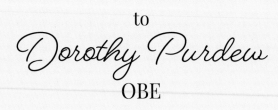

Dorothy Purdew

OBE

First published in Great Britain in 2023 by Aster,
an imprint of Octopus Publishing Group Ltd
Carmelite House
50 Victoria Embankment
London EC4Y 0DZ
www.octopusbooks.co.uk

An Hachette UK Company
www.hachette.co.uk

Distributed in the US by Hachette Book Group
1290 Avenue of the Americas
4th and 5th Floors
New York, NY 10104

Distributed in Canada by Canadian Manda Group
664 Annette St.
Toronto, Ontario, Canada M6S 2C8

Some recipes are specified for those following a
gluten-free or dairy-free diet. It is prudent to check
the labels of all pre-prepared ingredients for the
inclusion of any ingredients that may contain gluten
or dairy, as different brands may vary.

Champneys Henlow Ltd. asserts the moral right
to be identified as the author of this work.

ISBN 978 1 78325 597 9

A CIP catalogue record for this book is available
from the British Library.

Printed and bound in China.

10 9 8 7 6 5 4 3 2 1

Publisher: Stephanie Jackson
Editor: Lucy Bannell
Art Director: Nicky Collings
Photographer: Holly Farrier
Food Stylist: Holly Cowgill
Props Stylist: Rachel Vere
Senior Production Manager: Peter Hunt

For Champneys
Group Executive Chef: Christopher Cloonan
Wellbeing Director: Louise Day
Senior Nutritionist: Becki Hawkins
Brand Innovation Director: Kate Taylor

ASTER

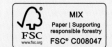

contents

Welcome
to Champneys

Trends come and go, but our unwavering commitment to encouraging wellness endures, and food is at the heart of that: the mainstay of a healthy lifestyle.

Champneys – the first resort of its kind in the UK – opened in 1925 as a health farm known as the Nature Cure Resort. It was born out of the ideals of visionary naturopath Stanley Lief, whose knowledge of the importance of a healthy diet, passion for holistic wellness and recognition of stress as bad for health can still be seen in our spas and their restaurants today. He was truly a man well ahead of his time.

Having been diagnosed with a seemingly incurable heart condition in 1890, a young Stanley sought – and found – a solution in a healthy diet and the practice of osteopathy. Self-cured by the age of 16, he went on to study naturopathy and, ultimately, founded Champneys in Tring. Pioneering the concepts of holistic health and naturopathy, the reputation of the resort grew, and patients visited from far and wide. Success was rapid and, lasting. These days, we welcome more than 100,000 guests every year. Some come to relax and de-stress, others to reconnect with friends and family, while many people visit us to reboot and to start new chapters in their lives. All of them get to enjoy the wonderful dishes prepared by our team of chefs.

Trends come and go, but our unwavering commitment to encouraging wellness endures, and food is at the heart of that: the mainstay of a healthy lifestyle.

We are often asked for our recipes, so we are delighted – through these pages – to now be able to bring you a mix of Champneys classic dishes as well as delicious creations from our latest menus.

This book is a celebration of our commitment to delicious natural ingredients. Hopefully, you will find new favourite dishes here. Most of the recipes are simple – you'll find great breakfasts for every mood, healthy snacks, indulgent yet nourishing desserts or spectacular salads – while others need a bit more time and effort to create a special lunch for friends, or an impressive dinner. You will discover that no dietary requirement is out of bounds. Whether you are vegan, gluten- or dairy-free, flexitarian, or even a hungry omnivore, there's a plethora of great dishes here for you.

Remember: once you have enjoyed your delicious meal, if you can, go for a walk and look at the world around you. Many things have changed since 1925, but the joy of taking time to enjoy a delicious and wholesome meal, followed by an inspiring walk, remains one of life's greatest simple pleasures. So take a look through this book and decide what you are going to cook today…

Here's to your good health!

The Champneys Team

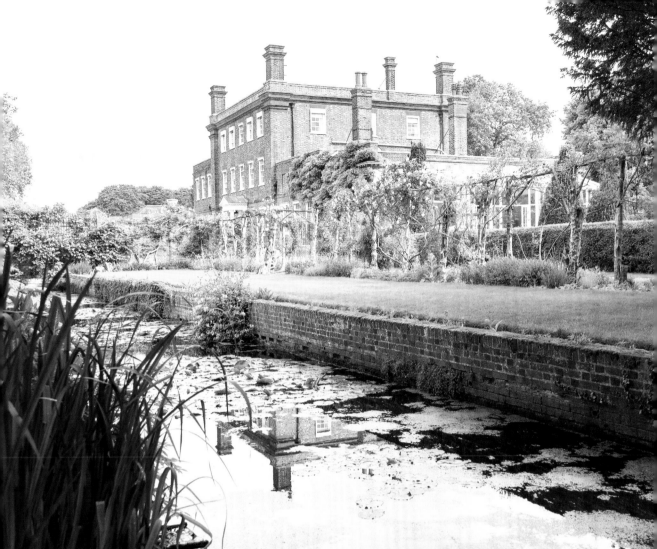

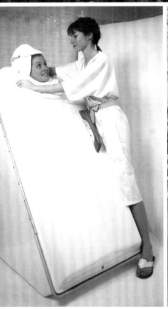

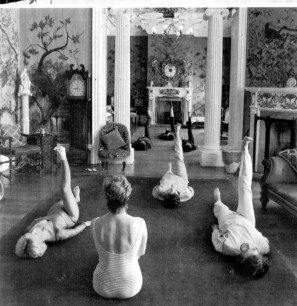

Clockwise from above:
Champneys Henlow
Grange, a beautiful
Georgian manor house
in Bedfordshire; the
famous Peacock Room
inside Champneys
Henlow Grange; a client
using a steam cabinet
at Champneys Henlow
Grange in the 1980s.

Food Philosophy
& the Champneys Plate

This visual approach makes life very easy and helps us enjoy a more balanced diet without missing out on foods we love.

Modern nutrition advice and food philosophy can be bewildering, even to the most seasoned cook. It can sometimes seem as though the experts are constantly changing their minds.

Every year, our chefs cook for thousands of guests and understand that everyone has their own individual relationship with food, as well as differing cultural and nutritional needs. We know that, during different life stages such as pregnancy, menopause, or even when training for sporting events such as triathlons, food requirements become temporarily different.

However, we firmly believe that everyone benefits from eating a colourful varied diet, with as many natural unprocessed foods as possible. Some of our recipes are devised using flexitarian principles: they are predominantly made with plants, but give you options about which protein to include, whether that is from pulses, meat, fish or eggs.

Eating more plant foods gives your body a rest from ultra-processed foods, inflammatory animal proteins and trans fats, as well as gluten, dairy and stressful stimulants such as refined sugar, alcohol and caffeine.

We recommend adding new foods to your diet rather than excluding any one food group, as it can be extremely beneficial for health. And we believe that, if a person's diet is less than ideal, this is more often due to poor eating habits than to 'bad' foods. Ensuring that you eat a balance of complementary whole foods – such as fruit, vegetables, pulses, legumes, nuts, seeds and unrefined grains – means you will fulfil all your macronutrient (protein, carbohydrate and fat) plus micronutrient (vitamin and mineral) requirements.

The Champneys plate removes any need to weigh portions or count calories. It shows you how to devise a healthy meal to promote sensible weight management, while ensuring you eat all your body's essential nutrients. This visual approach makes life very easy and helps us enjoy a more balanced diet without missing out on foods we love. Even if you don't have a Champneys plate, you can use the image of it, opposite, to remind yourself of the ideal balance of foods on your plate at home.

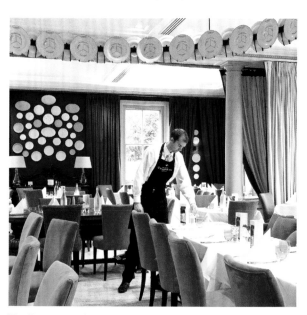

The Restaurant, Champneys Tring, Hertfordshire.

MODERATION

We all know the wisdom of maintaining portion sizes suited to our needs, but remember also to consider *how often* foods may find their way on to your plate.

BALANCE

The plate is perfect for finding the correct ratios of macronutrients – protein, carbohydrate and fat – whether putting a meal together or looking at your overall diet.

VARIETY

It's easy to fall into the trap of eating the same foods day after day. But different foods contain different nutrients, so we suggest eating as wide a variety of foods as possible.

NON-STARCHY VEGETABLES
UNLIMITED

such as: rocket
tomato
cucumber

onion
artichoke
broccoli

asparagus
mushroom
pepper

HEALTHY FATS
I TSP UNHEATED OIL
such as: extra virgin olive oil

HEALTHY PROTEINS
PALM-SIZED PORTION
such as: lean meat, white or oily fish, beans & lentils, nuts & seeds, tofu

FIBRE-RICH CARBOHYDRATES
FIST-SIZED PORTION
such as: brown rice, wholemeal bread & pasta, sweet potato, quinoa, oatcakes

The Champneys plate helps you:

- Maintain portion control • Understand food groups • Ensure a balance of nutrients • Eat more vegetables!
- Choose wholegrain, fibre-rich carbohydrates • Increase essential fats • Control calories and manage weight

Tips from Our Nutritionist

At Champneys we believe
in eating to thrive,
not to deprive.

This book aims to help you to enjoy nutritious and delicious recipes without being overwhelmed by science. We hope these tips will empower you to manage your own diet and health long term.

Not all foods are created equal

At Champneys we believe in eating to thrive, not to deprive. A well-balanced diet provides you with the energy and nutrients to do just that. We're all unique and so are our nutritional requirements. Individual responses to different foods can largely vary, too. This can be related to digestion, blood sugar response, metabolism and how our genes can shape our propensity to certain health risks. Ideally, we'd all have a personal nutritionist and chef to help plan meals, but, in the real world, a gradual change of habits, as suggested here, will be likely to support us all towards improved nutrition and health.

You need essential fats

We should limit animal fats and hydrogenated oils found in meat, dairy and ultra-processed foods and replace them with essential fats, especially omega 3. These fats are vital for cardiovascular health and our brains, but cannot be made in our bodies, so we must eat them.

For omega 3 – in which we are often deficient – flexitarians should turn to oily fish such as salmon, mackerel and trout, while plant-based eaters should incorporate flaxseed oil, walnuts, pumpkin seeds, algae and chia seeds. We don't tend to lack omega 6 as much, which is found in a wide variety of oils.

Eat protein with each meal or snack

Protein is essential for our bodies' cellular growth and repair. It forms the material for cells and organs and makes hormones, enzymes and antibodies. It helps stabilise blood sugar levels and keep us satisfied; it fills us up for longer, so we eat less. Try to eat a palm-sized portion at each meal.

Plant proteins – legumes, nuts and seeds – are generally lower in saturated fat and higher in fibre than animal equivalents, so are easier on digestion and less inflammatory. For a protein-rich snack, try an apple with nut butter, or houmous and oatcakes, or a blended vegetable and fruit smoothie containing a scoop of high-quality plant protein powder.

Healthy gut, healthy body

Our gut microbiome may influence our digestion, immune system, weight management and many other aspects of health. We can support the trillions of microorganisms in our gut by eating fermented foods every day, such as kefir, unpasteurised sauerkraut, kimchi and kombucha. Our gut may also link to our mental wellbeing and is sometimes termed our 'second brain', as the majority of serotonin production happens here. Serotonin is a neurotransmitter that supports our mood and emotions.

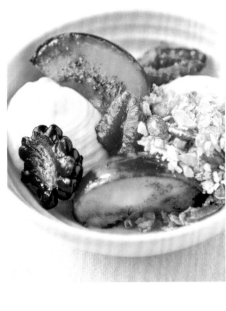

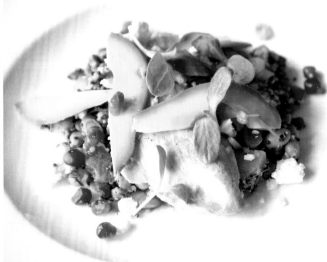

Our philosophy is simple: at Champneys, it's all about healthy, delicious and beautiful food.

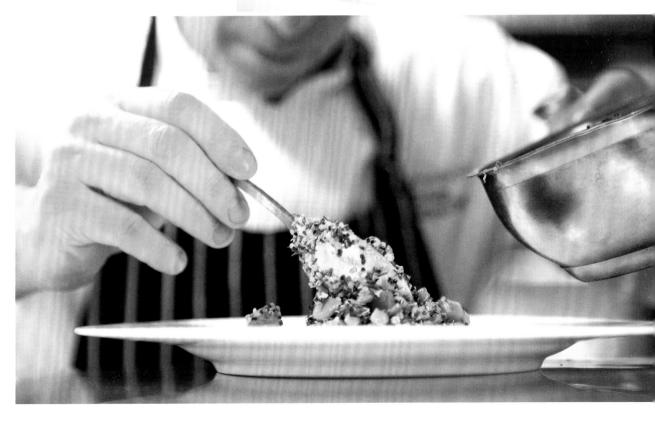

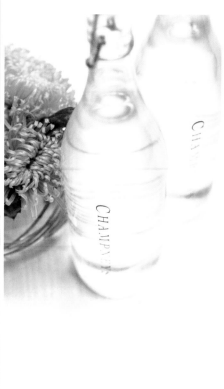

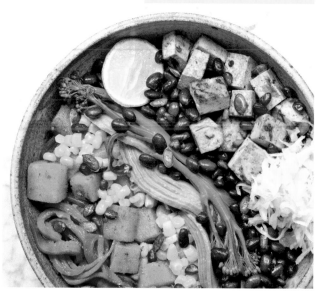

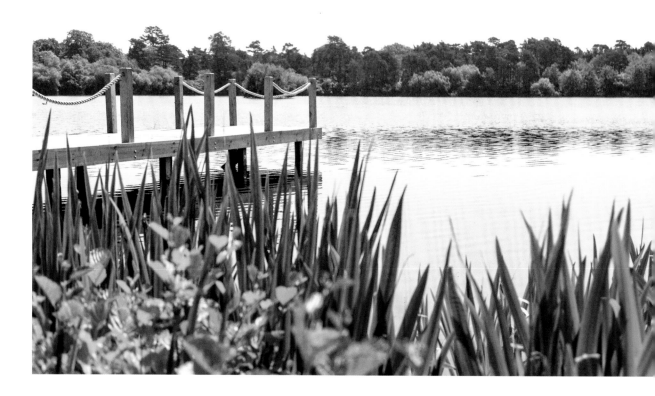

Plant-focused eating can help add low-calorie, nutrient-dense food to meals, snacks and desserts while leaving your good gut microbes thriving.

Put plants first... 30, to be exact!

For effective, sustainable health and weight management, plant-focused eating is a great way to go. It can help add low-calorie, nutrient-dense food to meals, snacks and desserts while leaving your good gut microbes thriving.

Research suggests that aiming for 30 different plants a week is a great target.

A 'rainbow' of fruits and vegetables offers wonderful preventative and protective health benefits, as they are rich in antioxidant nutrients such as vitamins A, C, E, zinc, selenium, plus a variety of fibres to support digestive health. So eat your way through those red, orange, yellow, green and purple plants to rack up your plant points. Dark green leafy vegetables and dark-coloured berries may be some of the most favourable in plant power potential.

Switch from white to brown

White carbohydrates – such as bread, pastries, pasta, rice and many breakfast cereals – are refined. During processing, they lose most of their fibre and nutrients. They provide bulk, but we're actually likely to absorb more calories from these foods. They only satisfy us temporarily, as they case a surge in our blood sugar levels, followed by a steep decline. This can very quickly leave us hungry, irritable and with cravings for more refined foods.

Riding this blood sugar rollercoaster also encourages weight gain, insulin resistance and long-term cardiovascular risks. So opt for wholegrain foods such as oats, brown rice, quinoa, wholemeal seeded bread and wholewheat pasta. These options are richer in fibre, protein, vitamins and minerals, particularly B vitamins. Their slow-release carbohydrates help stabilise blood sugar levels, energy and mood throughout the day. By keeping your blood sugar levels balanced, you will feel fuller for longer and reduce your cravings, discouraging weight gain.

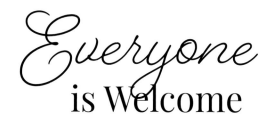

Everyone is Welcome

Our recipes are set out to be as helpful to you as possible, because the nutritional information of a portion of each dish is provided.

 We work hard at Champneys to ensure that all our guests, whatever their dietary requirements, get the same enjoyment out of our food. As you read through the book, you will see that recipes are marked 'vegan', 'vegetarian', 'gluten-free' or 'dairy-free'. Of the 103 recipes in these pages, 55 are vegan and another 19 vegetarian: that's nearly three-quarters of them. And some of the dishes can pivot from vegan to pescetarian, or from vegetarian to vegan; you will find details in the recipes about how to do that.

Our recipes are set out to be as helpful to you as possible, because the nutritional information of a portion of each dish is provided. There are broad national guidelines laid out about what the ratio of each macronutrient – protein, carbs and fats – should be in adult diets, but there are also a plethora of other guidelines for more specialist diets, such as lower carb, low calorie or low sugar. So knowing how much of each appear in the recipes helps us balance our daily eating to our own bespoke requirements.

We've listed some of the delicious recipes (see opposite) that will suit you, whatever your body needs.

A NOTE ON INGREDIENTS
Try to source the highest quality ingredients your budget allows. If you can, buy from a local farm shop, market, fishmonger or local butcher.

Fats and oils
For many years, sunflower or rapeseed oil was seen as more beneficial than butter and ghee, though research now suggests some seed oils should be avoided. And depending on whether the oil is refined or heated – and to what temperature – the advice changes again. In our recipes, we use olive oil and cold-pressed rapeseed oil (great for salads), vegetable oil (good for a high cooking temperature) and coconut oil (for cooking over low heat, or desserts). When we specify olive oil spray, we hope you will make you own: you can buy oil spray bottles, decant your preferred oil and spritz it to reduce the amount used and therefore a dish's fat and calorie content. We recommend you avoid commercial sprays, which add stabilisers and other ingredients.

When we went back to our archives, we found that the *Champneys Handbook of Nature Cure* (1962) advised cooking with an ounce of butter. Some would say that the advice has gone full circle. Whichever fat you decide to cook with, our philosophy is to use as little as possible.

Sugars and sweeteners
In our recipes, where possible we use the natural sweetness of ingredients such as fruit. However, when needed, we also use a mixture of honey, maple syrup and xylitol and only rarely sugar. Xylitol is a naturally occurring substance widely used as a sugar substitute, found in some fruits, vegetables and grains. It has been widely studied and there are reported health benefits for oral and dental health. If you prefer to use sugar, it can be substituted in the same exact quantities.

Recipes for Every Diet

breakfast

Lower carb

Avo scramble sundae
(see page 38)

Gluten-free

Champneys signature
soaked muesli
(see page 22)

Apple and cinnamon
overnight oats with pumpkin
seeds *(see page 27)*

Dairy-free

Cloud eggs with the best
baked beans
(see page 42)

Vegan

Banoffee chia breakfast pots
(see page 23)

Plant protein power
smoothie bowl
(see page 34)

lunch

Lower carb

Spinach, mozzarella and
caramelised pink grapefruit
salad *(see page 97)*

Roasted chicken breast,
cavolo nero, squash purée
and salsa verde
(see page 121)

Gluten-free

Coconut, coriander and lime
cauliflower rice salad
(see page 85)

Seafood and sweet potato
tikka masala
(see page 117)

Dairy-free

Champneys superfood
salad *(see page 76)*

Roasted sea bass, aubergine
caviar and corn salsa
(see page 114)

Vegan

Red rice and bean salad
with avocado and mango,
(see page 98)

Protein-packed tomato,
avocado, rocket and
onion salad
(see page 106)

dinner

Lower carb

Rainbow soul bowl
(see page 156)

Gluten-free

Grilled lamb cutlets,
quinoa salad, tzatziki
(see page 184)

Mexicana black bean
lettuce cups
(see page 154)

Dairy-free

Duck and bean burrito
with red cabbage and
pomegranate slaw
(see page 182)

Prawn and vegetable ramen
with ginger soy broth and
glass noodles *(see page 168)*

Vegan

Green lentil and sweet
potato cottage pie
(see page 152)

Tempeh chow mein with
buckwheat noodles and
peanuts *(see page 163)*

snacks and juices

Lower carb

Green spirulina shot
(see page 52)

Pomegranate hibiscus shot
(see page 52)

Edamame, mint and miso dip
(see page 66)

Gluten-free

Choco-nut protein power
shake *(see page 59)*

Sweet potato, smoked paprika
and white bean dip
(see page 66)

Dairy-free

Kick-start coconut coffee
smoothie *(see page 54)*

Black bean, coriander and
chilli dip *(see page 74)*

Vegan

Iced spiced golden coconut
latte *(see page 58)*

Beetroot and wasabi
houmous *(see page 71)*

sweet treats

Lower carb

Raspberry and lemon
cheesecake bliss balls
(see page 189)

Watermelon berry pizza
(see page 194)

Gluten-free

Salted caramel bliss balls
(see page 192)

Blueberry and lemon eton
mess *(see page 198)*

Dairy-free

Black Forest bliss balls
(see page 189)

Vegan tiramisu
(see page 214)

Vegan

Rocky road bliss balls
(see page 192)

Dark chocolate and
orange mousse
(see page 197)

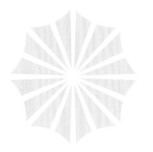

Breakfast

Champneys granola
with super seeds and berries

VEGETARIAN | GLUTEN-FREE | DAIRY-FREE

SERVES 4

2 teaspoons cold-pressed
    rapeseed oil
1 tablespoon agave syrup
1 teaspoon honey
1 teaspoon vanilla extract
120g oats (gluten-free)
20g sunflower seeds
20g pumpkin seeds
5g sesame seeds
10g mixed chopped nuts
10g whole flaxseed
15g desiccated coconut
20g dried chopped apricots
20g goji berries
finely grated zest of
    ½ orange
finely grated zest of
    ½ lemon

1 Preheat the oven to 170°C (150°C fan), Gas Mark 3½ with a baking tray inside to warm up.

2 Mix the oil, agave syrup, honey and vanilla in a large bowl. Tip in the next 6 ingredients and mix well.

3 Tip the granola on to the hot baking tray, spreading it out thinly to ensure it crisps up. Bake for 15 minutes.

4 Remove from the oven, mix in the coconut, apricots, goji berries and zests and bake for a further 15 minutes. Remove from the oven, turn out on to a cool tray and leave to firm up and cool completely.

_____ *Tip* _____

If you make this granola in a large batch (for instance, using ten times the ingredients here), it can be stored in an airtight container for up to one month.

NUTRITIONAL INFO PER SERVING

ENERGY 325 KCAL | FAT 15G | CARBS 33G | (OF WHICH SUGARS) 9.6G | PROTEIN 10G

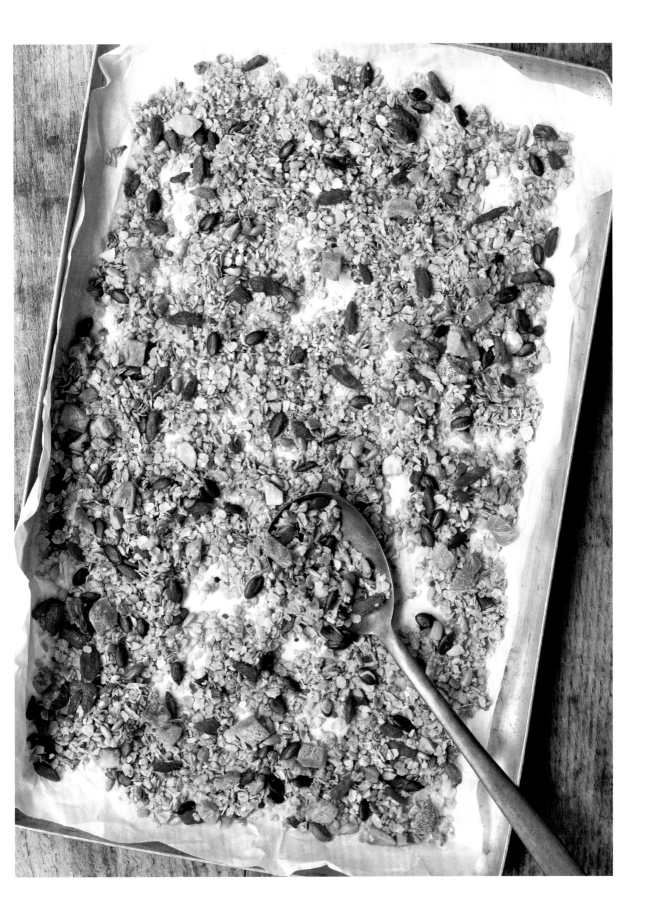

Kefir granola
berry parfait

VEGETARIAN | GLUTEN-FREE

SERVES 4

20g chia seeds
100ml rice milk
200g frozen mixed berries,
    defrosted
20ml maple syrup
200g kefir
60g granola (gluten-free, for
    homemade, see page 18)
fresh berries and mint
    leaves, to serve (optional)

1   Soak the chia seeds in the rice milk overnight; they should soak for a minimum of 8 hours. Defrost the berries, ready for the morning.

2   The next day, stir the maple syrup into the chia.

3   Now layer all the ingredients in 4 glass jars: start with the defrosted berries, with a little of their juice, then top with the chia mix. Next, divide the kefir between the pots, sprinkle on the granola and serve, topped with fresh berries and mint leaves, if you like.

NUTRITIONAL INFO PER SERVING

ENERGY 108 KCAL | FAT 2.9G | CARBS 15G | (OF WHICH SUGARS) 13G | PROTEIN 3.5G

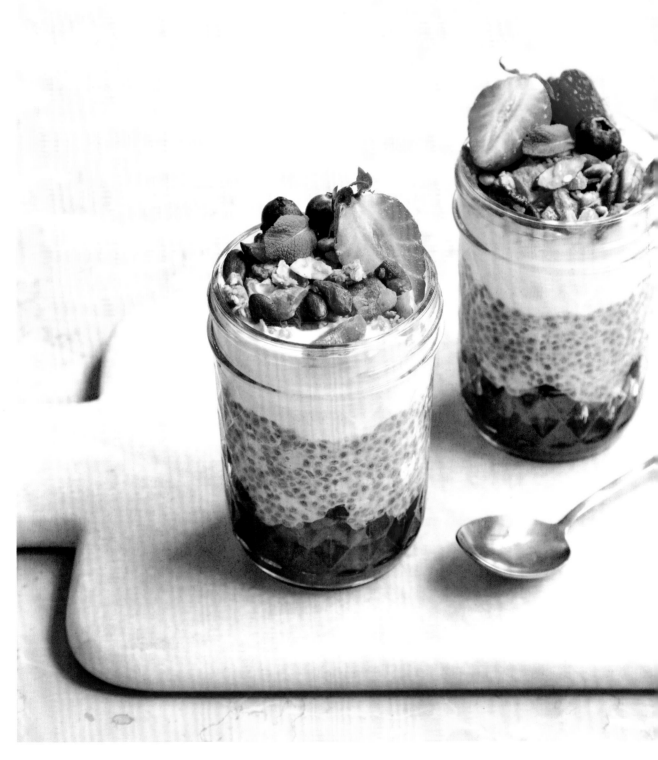

Champneys signature soaked muesli

VEGAN | GLUTEN-FREE | DAIRY-FREE

SERVES 4

120g oats (gluten-free)
25g dried cranberries
25g sultanas
30g hazelnuts, chopped
300ml unsweetened
    soya milk
30ml orange juice
60ml natural soya yoghurt
    (gluten-free)
½ apple
½ pear
fresh fruit, nuts and seeds
    to serve (optional)

1 Place all the dry ingredients in a bowl, stir in the soya milk, cover and leave the muesli to soak overnight in the fridge.

2 The next morning, stir in the orange juice and yoghurt. Peel and core the apple and pear and grate them into the muesli, mix well and serve, with fresh fruits, nuts and seeds, if you like.

Tip

This recipe can be adapted by adding other dried fruits and toasted sunflower or pumpkin seeds, or by using a different fruit juice.

NUTRITIONAL INFO PER SERVING

ENERGY 251 KCAL | FAT 8.8G | CARBS 36.5G | (OF WHICH SUGARS) 13.4G | PROTEIN 6.8G

Banoffee chia breakfast pots

VEGAN | GLUTEN-FREE | DAIRY-FREE

SERVES 4

60g chia seeds, ideally white
240g canned coconut milk
4 tablespoons water
1 teaspoon vanilla extract
8 teaspoons maple syrup
40g almond butter
25g dried banana chips
pinch of sea salt (we use
    pink Himalayan)

1 In a blender, mix the chia seeds with 210g of the coconut milk and the measured water. Add the vanilla and 4 teaspoons of the maple syrup, then refrigerate for at least 8 hours, ideally overnight, to allow the soluble fibre in the chia to swell and absorb the moisture and all the flavours.

2 Meanwhile, make the salted caramel banana mix. In a blender, mix the almond butter, remaining maple syrup, all but 4 of the best-looking banana chips and the salt. Pour in the remaining 30g coconut milk and blend to a smooth caramel.

3 When the chia mixture is ready, check the texture, as you may need to stir in a splash of water to loosen it to the desired consistency. Layer the pudding in 4 bowls or glasses with the salted caramel banana mixture. Decorate with the reserved banana chips and a final drizzle of the caramel mix, then serve.

Tip

White chia seeds can be tricky to get hold of, but if you can find them (online whole food stores are a good place to look), they avoid the chia mixture turning a little grey, which can happen if using the black chia seeds.

NUTRITIONAL INFO PER SERVING

ENERGY 238 KCAL | FAT 15G | CARBS 14G | (OF WHICH SUGARS) 10G | PROTEIN 7.3G

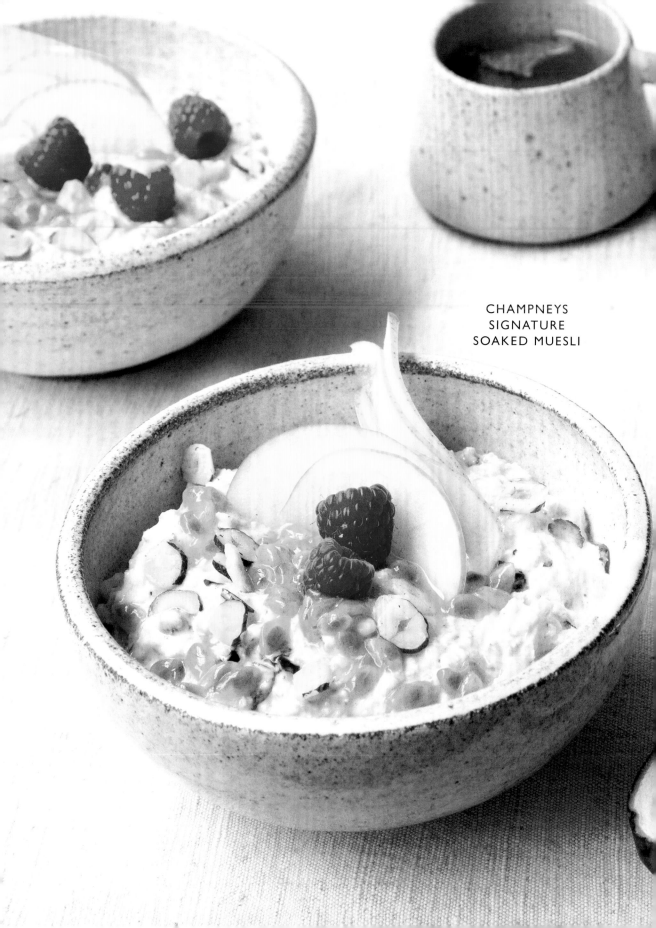

CHAMPNEYS
SIGNATURE
SOAKED MUESLI

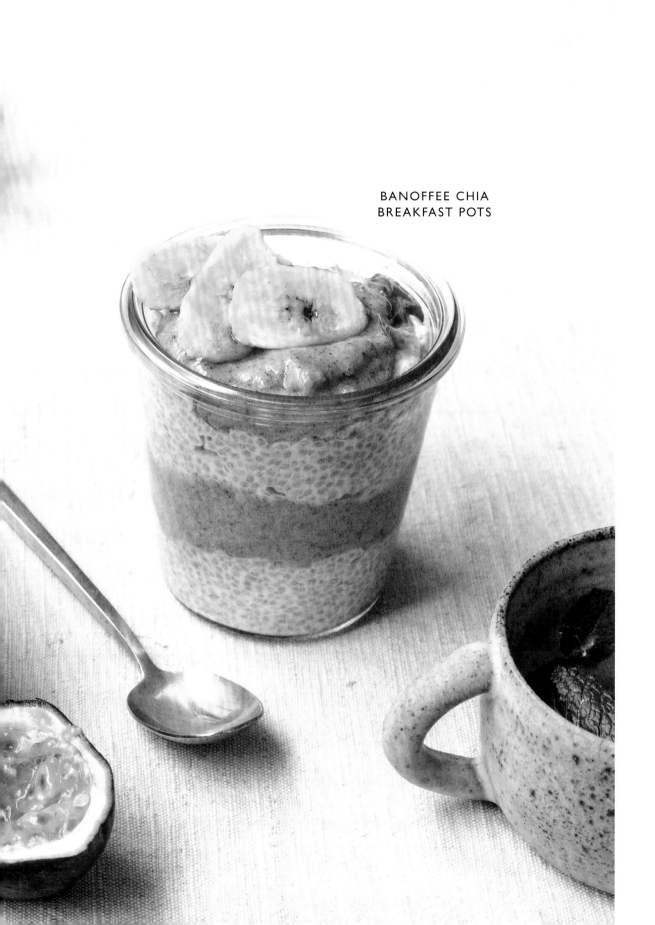

BANOFFEE CHIA
BREAKFAST POTS

Coconut, ginger
and turmeric protein porridge

VEGAN | GLUTEN-FREE | DAIRY-FREE

SERVES 2

100g oats (gluten-free)
200ml canned light
   coconut milk
200ml water
½ teaspoon ground
   turmeric
½ teaspoon ground ginger
1 tablespoon
   desiccated coconut

TO SERVE
(ALL OPTIONAL)
dairy-free yoghurt
   (gluten-free)
nuts
seeds
dried fruit

1   Put the oats, coconut milk, measured water, spices and desiccated coconut in a large saucepan and place it over a medium heat.

2   Bring to the boil, then reduce the heat and simmer, stirring, for around 10 minutes. Add a splash or so more water during the cooking time, if needed, to maintain a good consistency as the porridge thickens.

3   Serve with whichever toppings you like for an exotic twist, or leave the porridge plain.

Tip

Adjust the cooking time to achieve the consistency you favour. If you like your porridge to be a little sweeter, you could add 1 teaspoon maple syrup.

NUTRITIONAL INFO PER SERVING

ENERGY 359 KCAL | FAT 21.1G | CARBS 31.7G | (OF WHICH SUGARS) 2.6G | PROTEIN 7.7G

Apple and cinnamon overnight oats
with pumpkin seeds

VEGAN | GLUTEN-FREE | DAIRY-FREE

SERVES 4

80g oats (gluten-free)

80g chia seeds

600ml unsweetened
   almond milk

200ml water

2 teaspoons ground
   cinnamon

2 teaspoons vanilla extract

2 large apples (keep the
   skins on)

20g pumpkin seeds

1   Mix the oats and chia seeds in a large bowl with the almond milk, measured water, cinnamon and vanilla. Cover, then leave for at least 8 hours, but ideally overnight in the fridge.

2   The next morning, core the apples (keep the skins on), then grate or chop them and layer them in 4 bowls with the oat mixture.

3   Scatter with the pumpkin seeds, then serve.

____ *Tip* ____

We make our overnight oats gluten- and dairy-free to suit our guests' wide range of dietary requirements, but you could use regular oats and cow's milk instead, if you prefer.

NUTRITIONAL INFO PER SERVING

ENERGY 296 KCAL | FAT 12G | CARBS 30G | (OF WHICH SUGARS) 14G | PROTEIN 10G

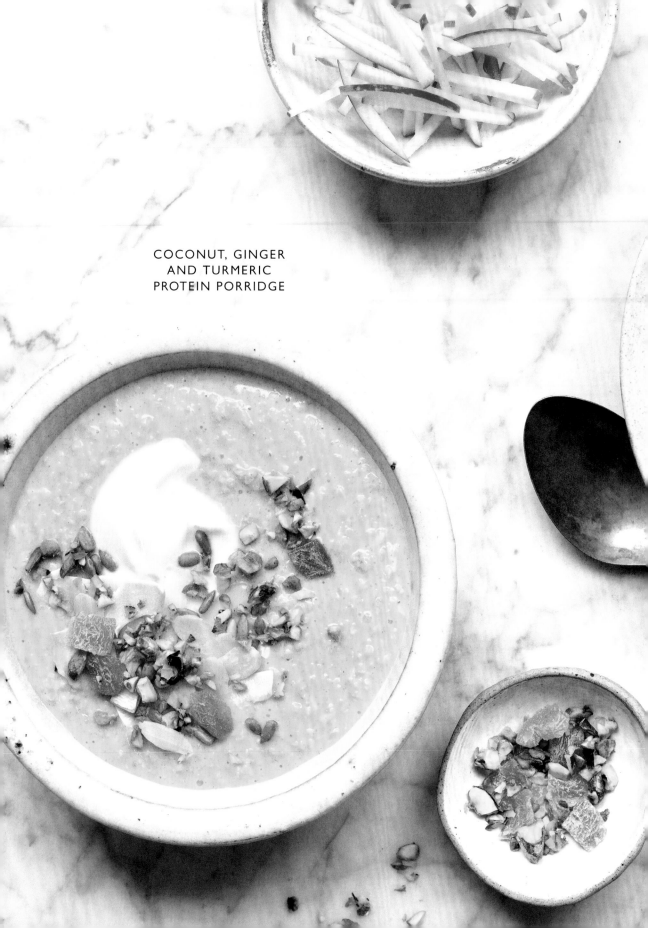

COCONUT, GINGER
AND TURMERIC
PROTEIN PORRIDGE

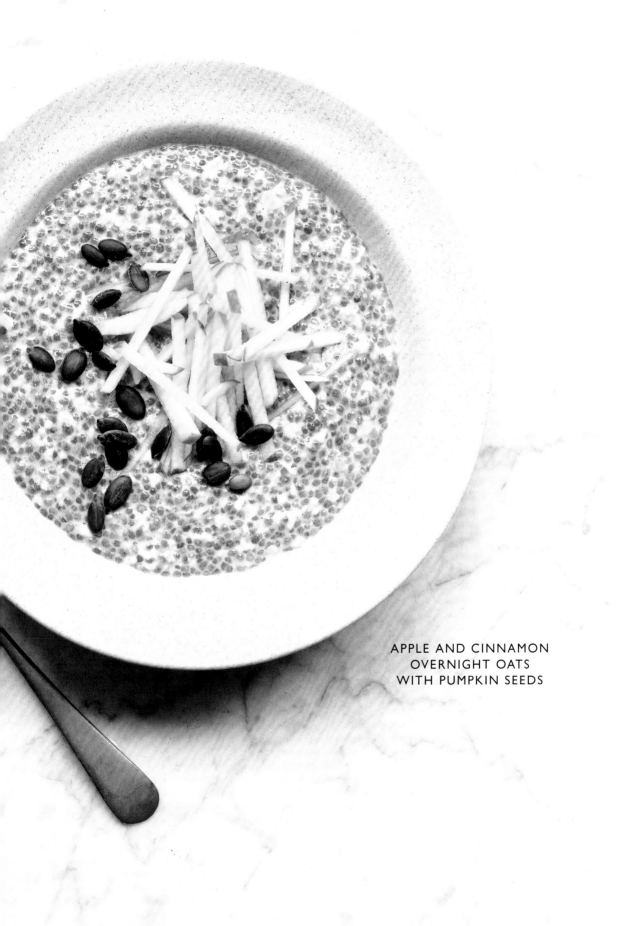

APPLE AND CINNAMON
OVERNIGHT OATS
WITH PUMPKIN SEEDS

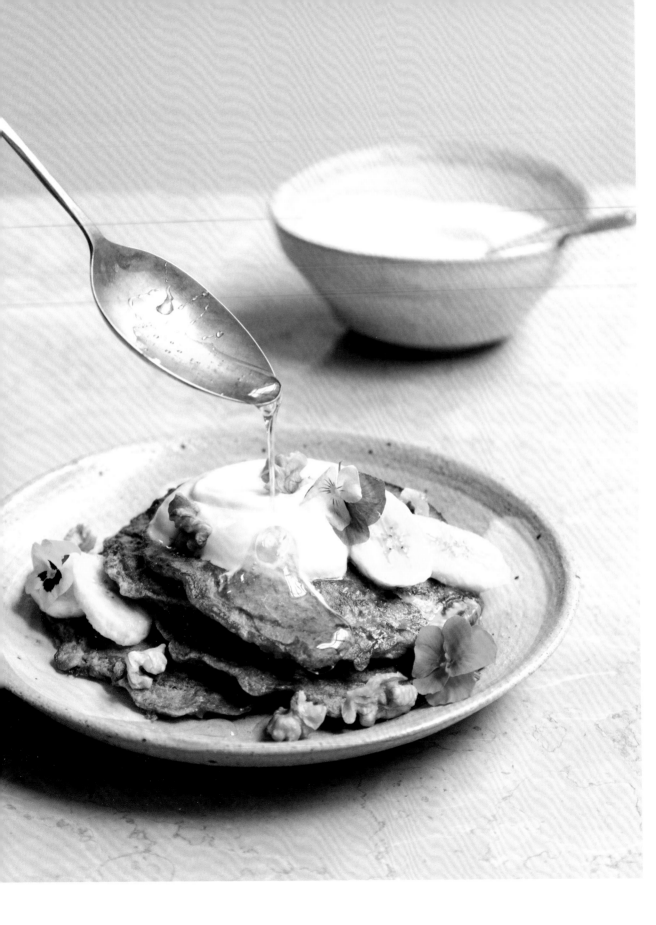

Banana walnut protein pancakes

VEGETARIAN | GLUTEN-FREE | DAIRY-FREE

SERVES 4 / MAKES 8

4 small bananas

4 medium eggs,
   lightly beaten

40g walnuts, chopped

4 teaspoons ground
   cinnamon

2 teaspoons vanilla extract

2 teaspoons coconut oil
   (we use raw organic
   extra-virgin)

1   Peel the bananas, mash them in a bowl and lightly beat in the eggs. Add the walnuts, cinnamon and vanilla and mix well.

2   Rub a frying pan with a little of the coconut oil and place it over a medium heat.

3   Pour in one-eighth of the mixture for each pancake and cook it for 3–4 minutes, then flip and cook the pancake on the other side for another 3–4 minutes. (You may have to cook them in batches.) Repeat to cook all the pancakes, then serve.

_____ *Tip* _____

For a smoother consistency, blitz the bananas and eggs in a blender. And for a super-indulgent breakfast, serve these with dairy-free Greek yoghurt, sliced bananas, a little honey and a few walnut halves (and even edible flowers, for a special occasion).

NUTRITIONAL INFO PER SERVING

ENERGY 265 KCAL | FAT 17G | CARBS 17G | (OF WHICH SUGARS) 15G | PROTEIN 9.9G

Spiced sweet potato pancake stack

VEGETARIAN | GLUTEN-FREE | DAIRY-FREE

SERVES 2 / MAKES 8

- 125g sweet potato (about 1 medium), scrubbed
- 2 medium eggs, lightly beaten
- 2 teaspoons ground cinnamon
- 2 teaspoons ground ginger
- 4 teaspoons coconut oil (we use raw organic extra-virgin)
- 200g dairy-free natural yoghurt (gluten-free)
- 200g banana, sliced
- 100g frozen mixed berries, defrosted
- 20g pumpkin seeds
- 20ml maple syrup

1 The day before you want the pancakes, preheat the oven to 200°C (180°C fan), Gas Mark 6 and bake the sweet potato, on a tray lined with foil (or the syrupy juices will ruin the tray), for 30–40 minutes, or until cooked through. Leave to cool in the fridge overnight.

2 The next day, remove the sweet potato flesh and purée until smooth.

3 In a bowl, mix the eggs and sweet potato together until fully combined. Stir in the cinnamon and ginger.

4 Heat the coconut oil in a frying pan over a medium heat, then spoon around 3 tablespoons of the mixture into the pan to make each pancake. Reduce the heat to medium-low and cook for 2–3 minutes. Flip and cook for another 2–3 minutes. (You may have to cook these in batches.) Repeat to cook all the pancakes.

5 Let the pancakes cool, then serve 4 in each stack, topped with the yoghurt, banana, berries and pumpkin seeds. Drizzle over the maple syrup and serve.

Tip

Cooking the sweet potato the night before and leaving it in the fridge overnight helps to reduce its moisture content, which in turn helps the pancake batter to bind together. This makes a great indulgent weekend breakfast

NUTRITIONAL INFO PER SERVING

ENERGY 542 KCAL | FAT 28.7G | CARBS 58.6G | (OF WHICH SUGARS) 39.5G | PROTEIN 12.7G

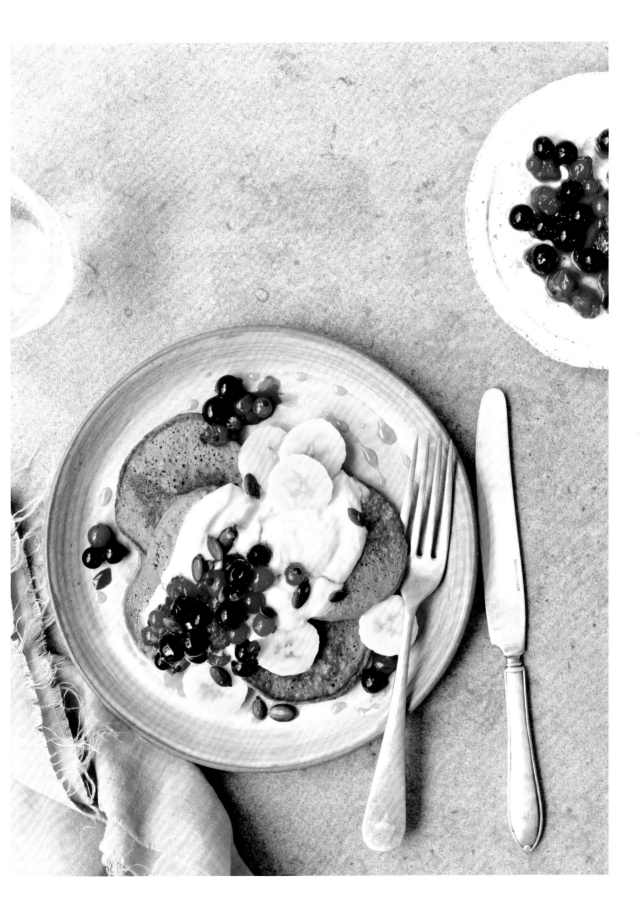

Plant protein power smoothie bowl

VEGAN | GLUTEN-FREE | DAIRY-FREE

SERVES 2

200g mango chunks,
    ideally frozen
2 large handfuls of fresh
    or frozen spinach
8 basil leaves
juice of 1 lime
1 tablespoon ground
    flaxseed
1 tablespoon coconut oil,
    melted (we use raw
    organic extra-virgin)
2 tablespoons unflavoured
    or vanilla flavour plant-
    based protein powder
    (gluten-free)
300ml plant-based milk,
    such as unsweetened
    almond or coconut
    drinking milk

TO SERVE
(ALL OPTIONAL)
fresh berries
toasted coconut flakes
toasted pumpkin or
    sunflower seeds
toasted nuts
edible flowers

1 Put all the ingredients into a high-powered blender and blend until smooth.

2 Pour into 2 bowls and top with berries, toasted seeds or nuts, or even edible flowers, to add crunch, boost nutrition and show off your creative flair!

NUTRITIONAL INFO PER SERVING

ENERGY 319 KCAL | FAT 14.3G | CARBS 30.3G | (OF WHICH SUGARS) 26.3G | PROTEIN 13.3G

Very berry beet smoothie bowl

VEGAN | GLUTEN-FREE | DAIRY-FREE

SERVES 2

2 carrots
150g mango
2 large cooked beetroots
100ml apple juice
100ml plant-based milk,
    such as unsweetened
    coconut drinking milk
100ml water

TO SERVE
(ALL OPTIONAL)
1 kiwi fruit
½ small banana
20g raspberries
20g blueberries
5g goji berries
10g whole flaxseeds
10g pumpkin seeds
10g flaked almonds
edible flowers

1 Peel the carrots and mango, roughly chop the beetroots and put them all into a high-powered blender or smoothie maker with the apple juice, milk and measured water.

2 Blend for 30–60 seconds, or until smooth. Divide the smoothie between 2 large shallow bowls and place slices of kiwi and banana in the centre. Decorate with the raspberries, blueberries, goji berries, flaxseeds, pumpkin seeds, flaked almonds and edible flowers, if you like.

Tip

It's easy to add vegetables to your breakfast if you choose to make a smoothie bowl. Try adding cucumber to a smoothie bowl flavoured with lime.

NUTRITIONAL INFO PER SERVING

ENERGY 323 KCAL | FAT 9G | CARBS 45G | (OF WHICH SUGARS) 39G | PROTEIN 8.1G

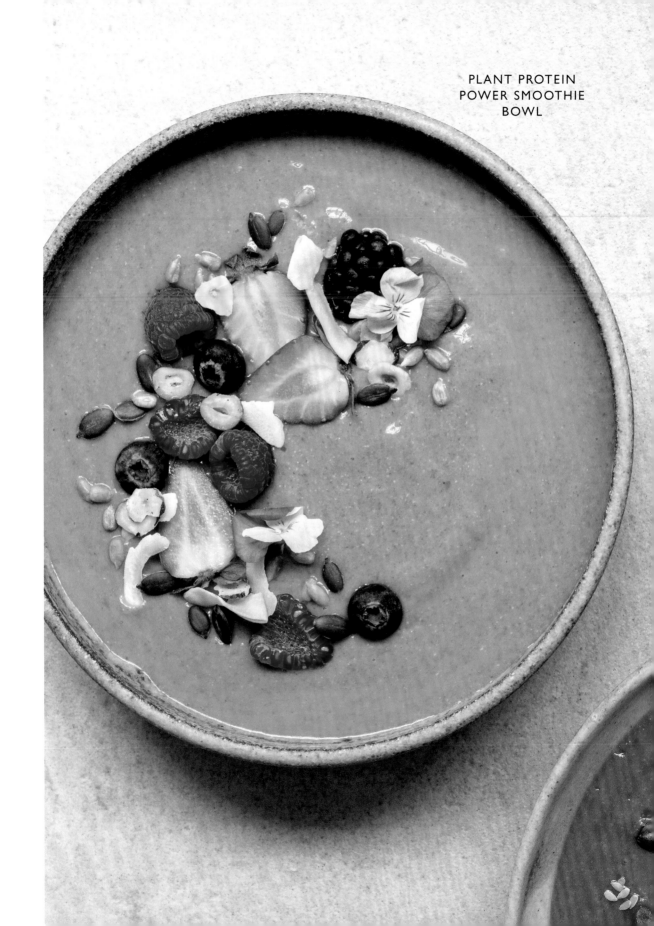

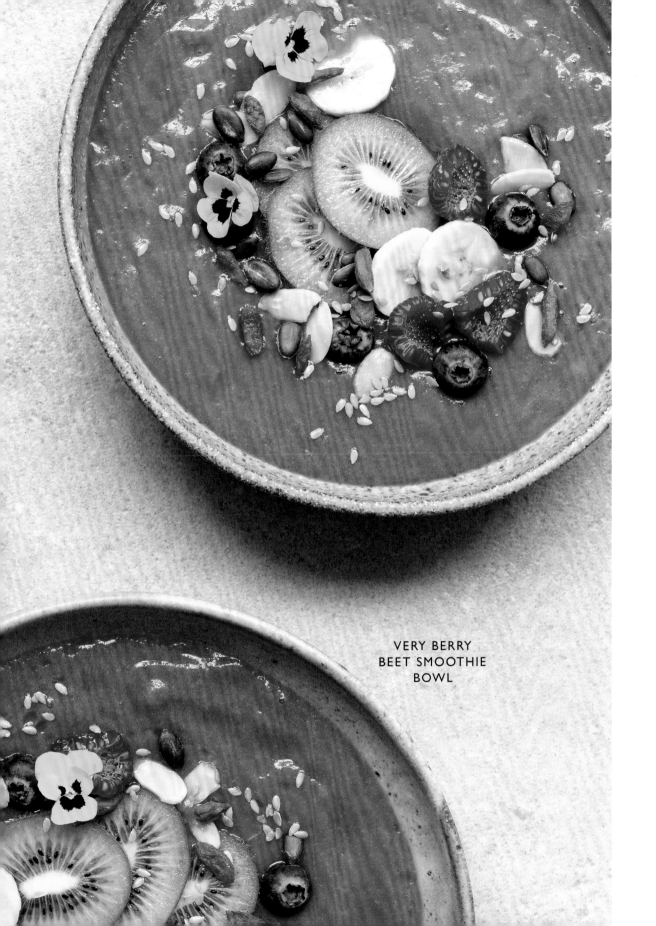

VERY BERRY
BEET SMOOTHIE
BOWL

Avo scramble sundae

VEGETARIAN | GLUTEN-FREE

SERVES 2

1 large avocado

1 teaspoon lemon juice

1 teaspoon chopped chives

1 teaspoon chopped
coriander leaves, plus
more to serve

2 medium tomatoes,
roughly chopped

1 teaspoon finely chopped
red onion

pinch of chilli flakes,
or to taste

2 eggs, plus 2 egg whites

2 tablespoons semi-
skimmed milk

½ teaspoon butter

olive oil spray

2 teaspoons pumpkin seeds

sea salt (we use pink
Himalayan) and cracked
black pepper

1   Halve the avocado and remove the stone. Remove the avocado flesh (a teaspoon is the easiest way to do this). Sprinkle some of the lemon juice over the avocado to stop browning and season with a little salt and pepper. Chop half into chunky pieces. Mash the other half in a bowl to a smoother consistency.

2   In a small bowl, mix the chives and coriander with the tomatoes, red onion, chilli flakes, a little seasoning and a few more drops of lemon juice.

3   Put the eggs and egg whites into a bowl or measuring jug. Add the milk and butter plus a little seasoning and beat until well combined.

4   Heat a medium frying pan and mist it lightly with olive oil spray. Add the egg mixture and stir continuously for 2–4 minutes until you reach your desired scrambled egg consistency.

5   Spoon one-quarter of the tomato mixture into 2 tall glass tumblers. Top with one-quarter of the scrambled egg. Add most of the chunky avocado, then divide the remaining tomato mixture between the glasses. Top with the remaining scrambled egg, then the smooth avocado, spreading it out for a neat finish.

6   Sprinkle the pumpkin seeds over, adding the remaining avocado and coriander leaves, then serve.

___ *Tip* ___

Remember that eggs keep on cooking for a little while once they're removed from the pan, so slightly under- rather than over-scramble them, for the perfect set.

NUTRITIONAL INFO PER SERVING

ENERGY 318 KCAL | FAT 24G | CARBS 7.3G | (OF WHICH SUGARS) 5.2G | PROTEIN 15G

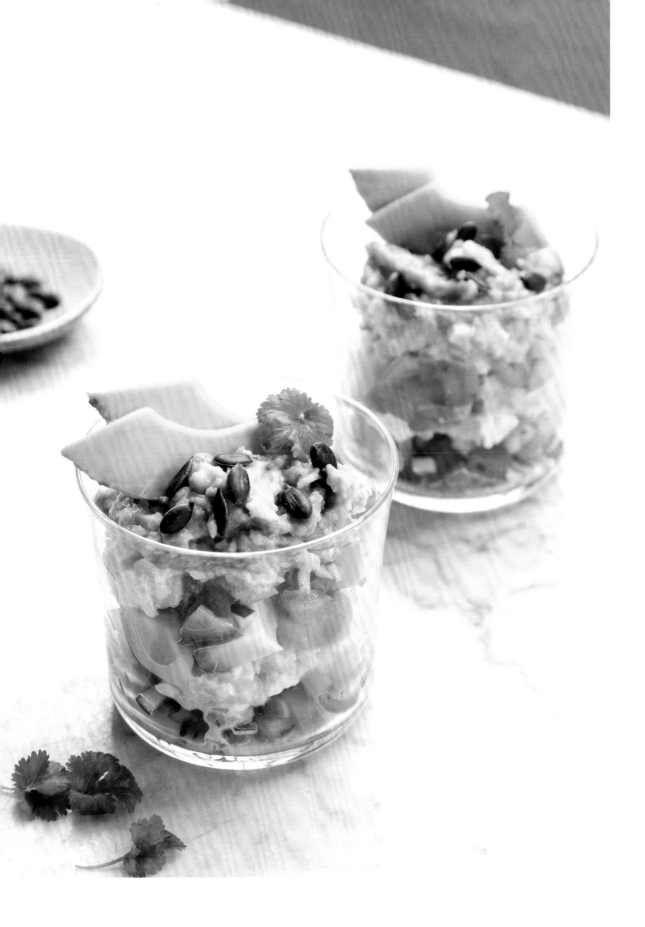

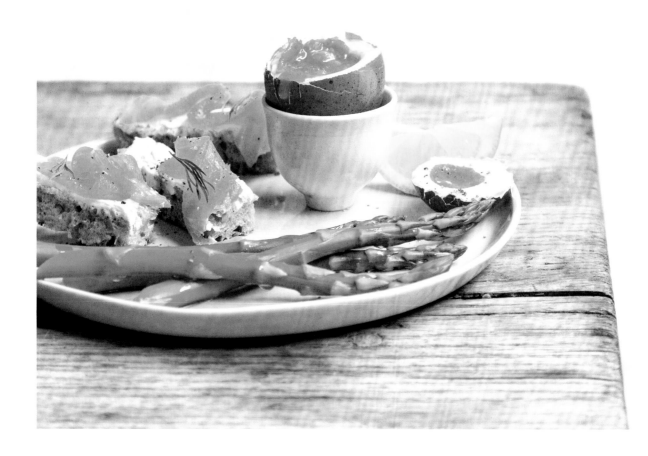

Dippy egg
with smoked salmon soldiers and asparagus

SERVES 2

2 medium eggs

12 asparagus spears

squeeze of lemon juice, plus
    lemon wedges to serve

50g smoked salmon

2 medium slices of seeded
    wholemeal bread

2 teaspoons cream cheese

sea salt (we use pink
    Himalayan) and freshly
    ground black pepper

1   Boil the eggs in gently simmering water for 4–5 minutes, or as you prefer for your perfect dippy egg.

2   Meanwhile, lightly steam the asparagus for around 4 minutes, then season.

3   Squeeze the lemon juice over the smoked salmon and asparagus.

4   Toast the bread, spread it with the cream cheese and top with the salmon, then cut it into soldiers.

5   Slice off the top of each egg and serve in an egg cup, with the asparagus, smoked salmon soldiers and lemon wedges on the side.

6   Use the smoked salmon soldiers and asparagus spears to dip into the egg.

___ *Tip* ___

Using seeded wholemeal toast boosts the fibre, protein and healthy fat content to make this breakfast really satisfying.

NUTRITIONAL INFO PER SERVING

ENERGY 292 KCAL | FAT 13G | CARBS 20G | (OF WHICH SUGARS) 2.4G | PROTEIN 20G

Cloud eggs
with the best baked beans

VEGETARIAN | DAIRY-FREE

SERVES 2

FOR THE BEANS
1 teaspoon olive oil
1 red onion, finely chopped
1 red pepper, finely chopped
400g can of haricot beans
200g canned kidney beans,
    drained weight
200g canned chopped
    tomatoes
3 tablespoons tomato
    ketchup
1 tablespoon maple syrup
1 tablespoon apple
    cider vinegar
1 teaspoon smoked paprika
½ teaspoon chipotle
    chilli flakes
Tabasco sauce, to taste

FOR THE EGGS
AND TOAST
2 medium eggs, separated
2 medium slices of seeded
    wholemeal bread
handful of chopped parsley
    leaves

1 To make the beans, heat the oil in a sauté pan and sauté the onion and pepper until softened. Add the beans, tomatoes and all the remaining ingredients and bring to a simmer. Let simmer for 10 minutes to thicken the mixture slightly and allow the flavours to combine.

2 Meanwhile, preheat the oven to 200°C (180°C fan), Gas Mark 6.

3 Whisk the egg whites until stiff, then place them – in 2 piles – on a baking tray lined with baking parchment, making a well in the middle of each pile, for the yolks.

4 Bake for 3 minutes.

5 Carefully tip an egg yolk into each nest of white, then return the tray to the oven and cook for a further 2 minutes.

6 Meanwhile, toast the bread.

7 Top each toast with beans and a cloud egg, then scatter with parsley and serve.

Tip

Eating more pulses is a healthy way to include plant proteins in your diet. It's a good move both for our bodies and for the planet.

NUTRITIONAL INFO PER SERVING

ENERGY 301 KCAL | FAT 8.9G | CARBS 26.5G | (OF WHICH SUGARS) 6.2G | PROTEIN 18.3G

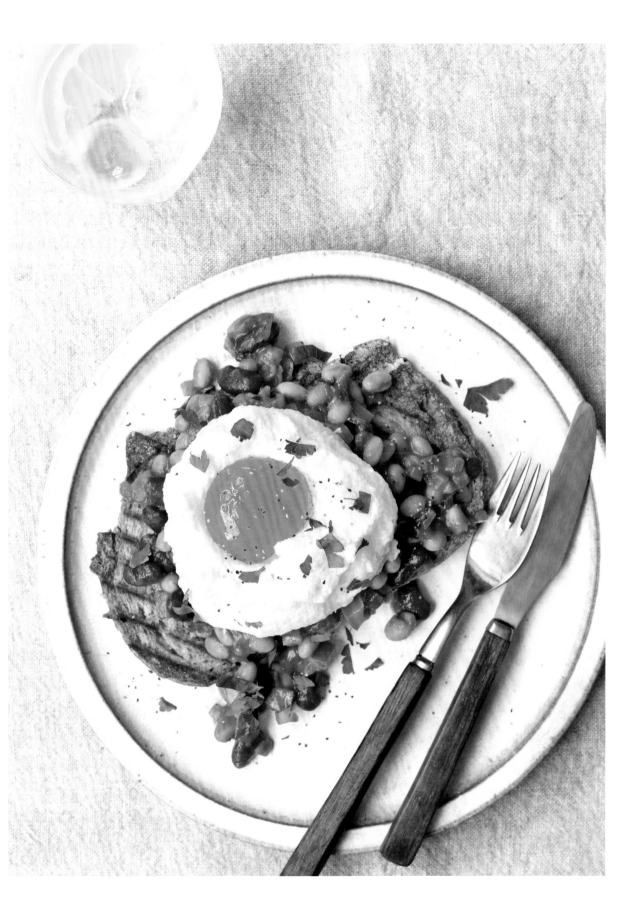

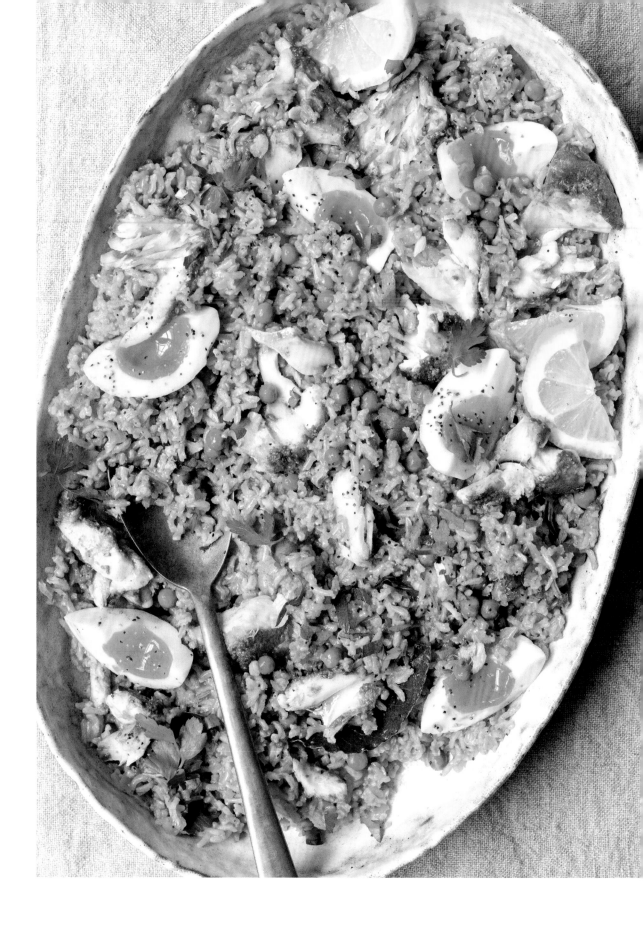

Modern masala kedgeree
with smoked haddock and herbs

SERVES 4

10g butter
1 small onion, finely
    chopped
½ teaspoon curry powder
    (gluten-free)
½ teaspoon ground
    turmeric
pinch of ground cinnamon
1 fresh or dried bay leaf
200g brown basmati rice
750ml vegetable stock
    (gluten-free)
250g smoked haddock fillet,
    skinned
1 tablespoon masala paste
    (gluten-free)
2 eggs
80g frozen peas, defrosted
2 tablespoons chopped
    parsley leaves
sea salt (we use pink
    Himalayan) and freshly
    ground black pepper
lemon wedges, to serve

1   Melt the butter in a large saucepan, add the onion and cook it gently over a medium heat for 5 minutes, until softened but not browned. Stir in the ground spices and bay, then cook for 1 minute.

2   Tip in the rice and stir until it is well coated in the spicy butter. Pour in the stock, season with salt and bring to the boil, stirring once to release any rice from the base of the pan.

3   Cover with a close-fitting lid, reduce the heat to low and leave to cook very gently for 20 minutes, or until the rice is cooked.

4   Meanwhile, preheat the oven to 200°C (180°C fan), Gas Mark 6. Coat the fish with the masala paste and place on a baking sheet. Bake for 8–10 minutes, until just cooked. Lift it out on to a plate and leave until cool enough to handle.

5   Bring a saucepan of water to the boil, then boil the eggs for 6–7 minutes for beautiful soft yolks.

6   Flake the fish, discarding any bones. Drain the eggs, cool slightly, then peel and carefully quarter.

7   Uncover the rice and remove the bay. Gently fork in the fish, eggs and peas, cover and return to the heat for 2–3 minutes, or until the fish has heated through completely, being careful to keep it in large chunks.

8   Gently stir in almost all the parsley and season to taste. Serve in shallow dishes with lemon wedges, scattered with the remaining parsley.

NUTRITIONAL INFO PER SERVING

ENERGY 312 KCAL | FAT 7.3G | CARBS 43.3G | (OF WHICH SUGARS) 2.8G | PROTEIN 20.0G

Mediterranean breakfast frittata

VEGETARIAN | GLUTEN-FREE

SERVES 2

2 medium eggs, plus
    4 medium egg whites
2 teaspoons olive oil
1 garlic clove, crushed
¼ onion, finely chopped
150g mushrooms,
    finely sliced
100g spinach, washed
100g cherry tomatoes,
    halved
small handful of herb leaves,
    such as parsley and chives
60g feta cheese (vegetarian)
handful of black olives
sea salt (we use pink
    Himalayan) and freshly
    ground black pepper

TO SERVE
(OPTIONAL)
rocket leaves
sliced tomatoes

1 Preheat the grill to medium-high.

2 Lightly beat the eggs and egg whites in a bowl.

3 Heat a medium ovenproof frying pan over a medium heat with the oil. Sauté the garlic for 1 minute, then add the vegetables, seasoning with salt and pepper and adding the herbs. Sauté for 3–4 minutes.

4 Pour the egg mixture over the vegetables, covering them evenly, then crumble over the feta and scatter with the olives. Cook the frittata for 3–4 minutes until the egg is partly set.

5 Finish cooking under the grill for 6–8 minutes, until the top of the frittata is set and slightly golden. Leave to cool slightly, then serve, with rocket and tomatoes for a burst of colour and goodness, if you like.

Tip

Using this combination of whole eggs and egg whites helps to limit the fat and calories, while still maximising the protein, to give you a really satisfying start to the day. If you'd rather use whole eggs, you will need six.

NUTRITIONAL INFO PER SERVING

ENERGY 272 KCAL | FAT 19G | CARBS 4.2G | (OF WHICH SUGARS) 1.6G | PROTEIN 22.5G

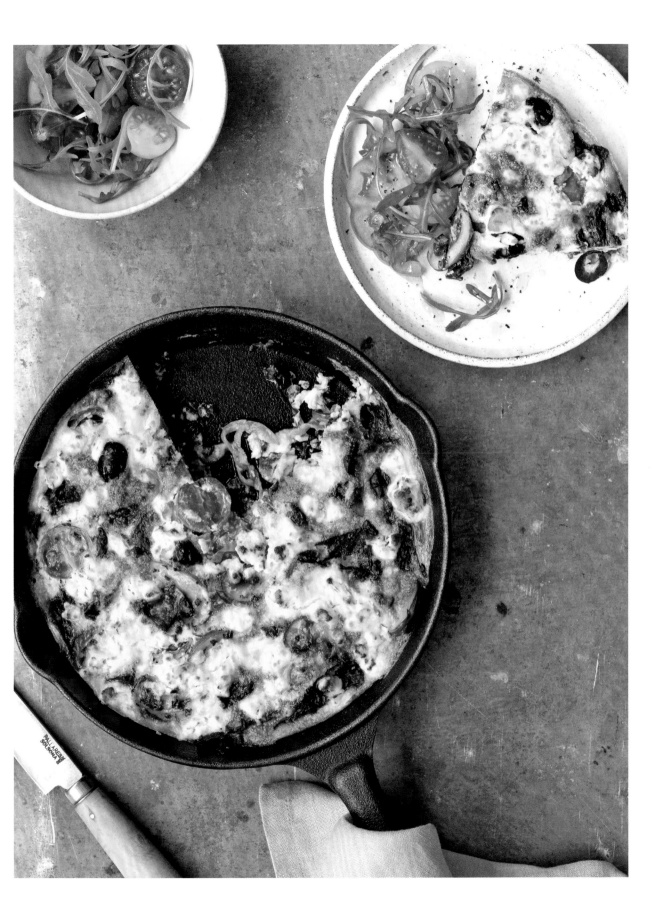

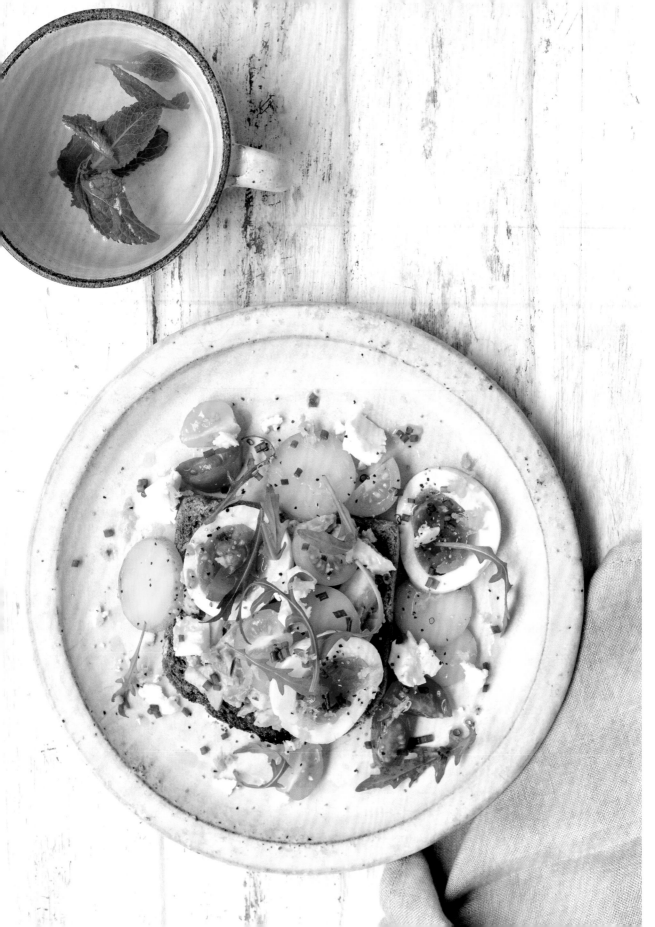

Stephen's balanced breakfast

VEGETARIAN | DAIRY-FREE

SERVES 2

150g baby new potatoes
2 medium eggs
2 x 40g slices of sourdough
    rye bread
1 medium avocado
20g vegan cream cheese
finely grated zest and juice
    of ½ lemon
finely chopped chives
30g vegan Greek-style
    cheese, cut into cubes
40g rocket leaves
100g cherry tomatoes,
    halved or quartered
1 teaspoon extra-virgin
    olive oil
sea salt (we use pink
    Himalayan) and freshly
    ground black pepper

1   Steam the baby potatoes for 5–6 minutes until soft, then slice them.

2   Boil the eggs for 5–6 minutes, or to your liking, then slice those, too.

3   Toast the bread. Peel the avocado, remove the stone and mix the flesh in a small bowl with the vegan cream cheese. Use this mixture to top the toasts, then season with most of the lemon zest and juice, most of the chives, salt and pepper.

4   Arrange over the sliced egg and baby potatoes.

5   Scatter the vegan Greek-style cheese, rocket leaves and cherry tomatoes on top, to dress the dish and add colour, then drizzle over the olive oil.

6   Scatter with more lemon zest and juice and chives, then serve.

_____ *Tip* _____

This recipe was created by Champneys owner Stephen Purdew, and is inspired by the food served at an Alpine health spa.

NUTRITIONAL INFO PER SERVING

ENERGY 307 KCAL | FAT 14G | CARBS 29.4G | (OF WHICH SUGARS) 3.1G | PROTEIN 13.7G

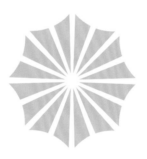

Juice Shots & Blended Drinks

Green
spirulina shot

VEGAN | GLUTEN-FREE | DAIRY-FREE

SERVES 4

2 kiwi fruits
juice of ½ lime
80g spinach
2 celery sticks
1 teaspoon spirulina powder
  (gluten-free)

1 Juice the first 4 ingredients in a juicer and mix well with the spirulina.

2 Chill, shake well to revive the drink and avoid separation, then serve in shot glasses.

Tip

To make this into a long drink, use the entire recipe for each serving, blending in a dash of water and ice.

NUTRITIONAL INFO PER SERVING

ENERGY 24 KCAL | FAT 0.5G | CARBS 2.8G | (OF WHICH SUGARS) 2.0G | PROTEIN 1.6G

Pomegranate
hibiscus shot

VEGAN | GLUTEN-FREE | DAIRY-FREE

SERVES 4

1 hibiscus tea bag
100ml freshly boiled water
100ml pure pomegranate
  juice (see tip, right)
4 mint leaves, chopped
juice of ½ lime

1 Steep the hibiscus tea bag in the boiling water for 3 minutes. Leave to cool, then remove the tea bag.

2 Combine all the ingredients together and stir.

3 Chill, then serve in shot glasses, shaking well before serving to revive the drink and avoid separation.

Tip

Use pure pomegranate juice here rather than 'juice drink', which has often been diluted and contains sugar or artificial sweeteners. Juicing the whole fruit yourself is an easy way to get it.

NUTRITIONAL INFO PER SERVING

ENERGY 34 KCAL | FAT 0G | CARBS 3.3G | (OF WHICH SUGARS) 2.8G | PROTEIN 0G

Lemon and ginger shot

with apple cider vinegar

VEGAN | GLUTEN-FREE | DAIRY-FREE

SERVES 2

1 apple
20g fresh root ginger, peeled
40ml coconut water
2 teaspoons lemon juice
1 teaspoon apple cider vinegar
   (see tip, below)
½ teaspoon ground turmeric
¼ teaspoon freshly ground black pepper

1   Peeling the apple is optional, depending on what works best in your juicer. Put the apple and ginger through a high-powered juicer. Combine this with the remaining ingredients and blend well until they all come together as one.

2   Chill, then serve in shot glasses, shaking well before serving to revive the drink and avoid separation.

_____ *Tip* _____

Apple cider vinegar is made by fermenting the sugar from apples. This turns them into acetic acid, a main ingredient in vinegar that may account for its health benefits.

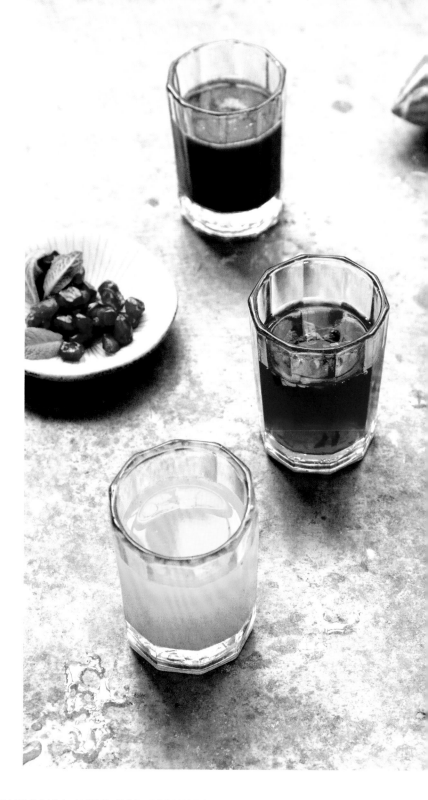

NUTRITIONAL INFO PER SERVING

ENERGY 51 KCAL | FAT 0.5G | CARBS 10G | (OF WHICH SUGARS) 8.1G | PROTEIN 0.7G

Pineapple and turmeric tropical smoothie

VEGAN | GLUTEN-FREE | DAIRY-FREE

SERVES 2

200g pineapple
½ medium banana
juice of ½ lime
300ml unsweetened
  coconut water
1 teaspoon coconut oil,
  melted

1 teaspoon ground
  turmeric, or finely grated
  fresh turmeric
ice
pinch of freshly ground
  black pepper

1   Place all the ingredients in a high-powered blender or smoothie maker and blend for around 1 minute, or until smooth. You may want to add some ice during the process if your blender can crush it, or serve over ice.

NUTRITIONAL INFO PER SERVING

ENERGY 166 KCAL | FAT 5.3G | CARBS 24G | (OF WHICH SUGARS) 22G | PROTEIN 1.5G

Kick-start coconut coffee smoothie

VEGAN | GLUTEN-FREE | DAIRY-FREE

SERVES 2

400ml freshly brewed
  coffee, cooled
100ml canned coconut milk
1 tablespoon coconut oil,
  melted (we use raw
  organic extra-virgin)
2 teaspoons xylitol

1 teaspoon vanilla extract
ice

1   Place all the ingredients in a high-powered blender or smoothie maker and blend for around 1 minute until smooth. You may want to add some ice during the process if your blender can crush it, or serve over ice.

NUTRITIONAL INFO PER SERVING

ENERGY 225 KCAL | FAT 22G | CARBS 6.7G | (OF WHICH SUGARS) 0.8G | PROTEIN 0.8G

Minted cucumber-lime matcha smoothie

VEGAN | GLUTEN-FREE | DAIRY-FREE

SERVES 2

1 teaspoon matcha green
  tea powder
300ml freshly boiled water
finely grated zest and
  flesh of 1 lime, plus lime
  wedges to serve
4 mint leaves, plus
  2 mint sprigs to serve

10g spinach
¼ cucumber
1 green apple, cored
2 teaspoons agave syrup
ice

1 Put the matcha powder into a cup with the boiling water. Whisk well and let it steep for 5 minutes, then leave to cool.

2 Blend the lime flesh, a little lime zest, the mint, spinach, cucumber and apple in a blender or smoothie maker, with the matcha and agave syrup.

3 Pour into 2 glasses over ice, or add ice during blending if your blender can crush it. Decorate each with a lime wedge and mint sprig.

NUTRITIONAL INFO PER SERVING

ENERGY 61 KCAL | FAT 0.5G | CARBS 12G | (OF WHICH SUGARS) 7.6G | PROTEIN 1.3G

Spicy mango and carrot smoothie

VEGAN | GLUTEN-FREE | DAIRY-FREE

SERVES 2

2 carrots, scrubbed
150ml coconut water
150ml water
1 mango, peeled and chopped
1 apple, skin on, chopped
2 teaspoons lemon juice
10g fresh root ginger, peeled
¼ teaspoon cinnamon
¼ teaspoon cayenne pepper

1 Top and tail the carrots (peeling is optional dependent on your blender), then roughly chop.

2 Place all the ingredients in a high-powered blender or smoothis maker and blend to the desired consistency. You may want to add some ice during the process if your blender can crush it, or serve over ice, to chill.

Tip

A serving of this smoothie – if you are able to leave all the skins on the fruit and vegetables – provides nearly 10g fibre. That's around one-third of an adult's recommended daily intake.

NUTRITIONAL INFO PER SERVING

ENERGY 164 KCAL | FAT 1.7G | CARBS 37.3G | (OF WHICH SUGARS) 35.5G | PROTEIN 2.2G

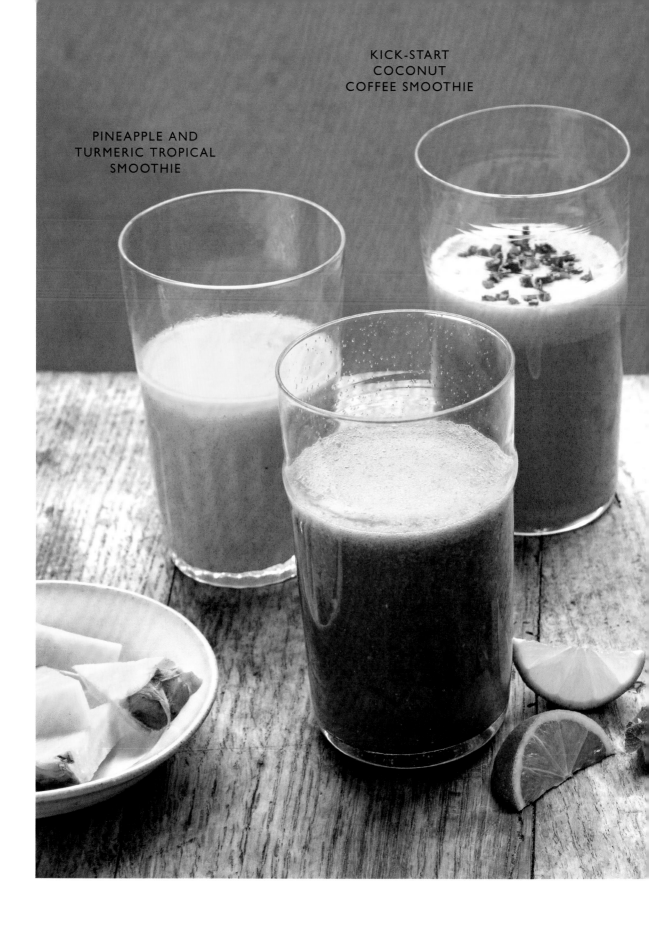

PINEAPPLE AND
TURMERIC TROPICAL
SMOOTHIE

KICK-START
COCONUT
COFFEE SMOOTHIE

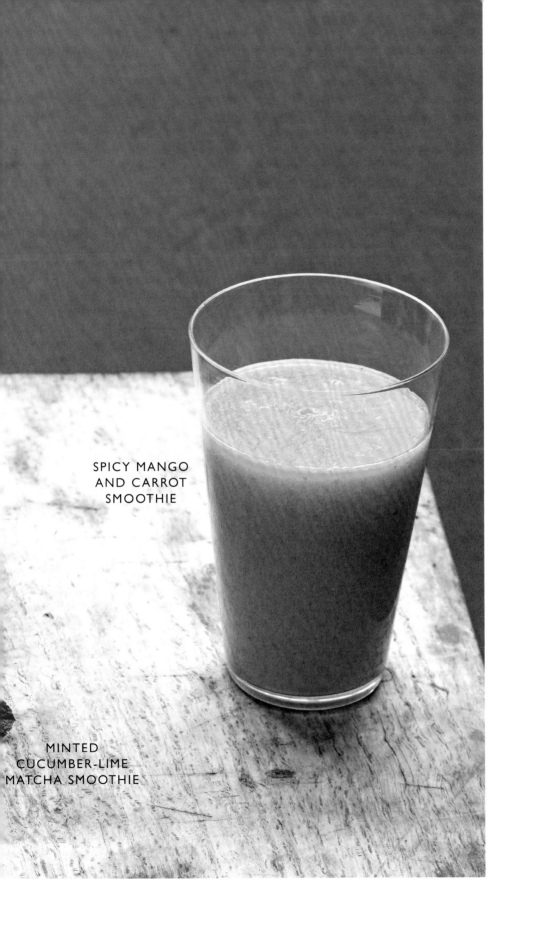

SPICY MANGO
AND CARROT
SMOOTHIE

MINTED
CUCUMBER-LIME
MATCHA SMOOTHIE

Iced spiced golden coconut latte

VEGAN | GLUTEN-FREE | DAIRY-FREE

SERVES 2

400ml unsweetened
    coconut milk drink
4 tablespoons canned
    coconut milk
1 tablespoon maple syrup
2 tablespoons xylitol
1 heaped teaspoon ground
    turmeric, plus more
    (optional) to serve
½ teaspoon ground
    cinnamon, plus more
    (optional) to serve
½ teaspoon ground ginger
¼ teaspoon freshly ground
    black pepper
¼ teaspoon ground
    cardamom seeds
ice
desiccated coconut, to
    serve (optional)

1   Blend all the ingredients in a high-powered blender for 1 minute until well combined, light and frothy. Ensure it's shaken well, to avoid the spices separating before serving. You may want to add some ice during the process if your blender can crush it, or serve over ice, to chill.

2   If you like, serve sprinkled with turmeric, cinnamon and/or desiccated coconut.

Tip

Try to use a mixture of both the liquid and solid parts of the canned coconut, for a really creamy and decadent drink.

NUTRITIONAL INFO PER SERVING

ENERGY 161 KCAL | FAT 7.4G | CARBS 27G | (OF WHICH SUGARS) 10G | PROTEIN 0.8G

Choco-nut protein power shake

VEGAN | GLUTEN-FREE | DAIRY-FREE

SERVES 2

1 tablespoon chia seeds

2 bananas

200ml unsweetened
   soya milk

200ml water

40g hazelnuts, plus more
   (optional) to serve

2 tablespoons cacao powder
   (gluten-free)

1 tablespoon maple syrup

1 tablespoon hazelnut
   butter

ice

pinch of sea salt

cacao nibs, to serve
   (optional)

1   The night before you want your shake, for the
smoothest drink possible, put the chia seeds into
a small bowl, cover with water, then chill for at least
8 hours, but ideally overnight. Drain the chia,
discarding the soaking liquid.

2   Place all the ingredients in a high-powered blender
and blend to your desired consistency. You may want
to add some ice during the process if your blender can
crush it, or serve over ice, to chill. Sprinkle with cacao
nibs and hazelnuts, if you like.

NUTRITIONAL INFO PER SERVING

ENERGY 405 KCAL | FAT 17G | CARBS 31G | (OF WHICH SUGARS) 26G | PROTEIN 14G

Blueberry, banana and kefir power shake

VEGETARIAN | GLUTEN-FREE

SERVES 2

200g frozen sliced banana

100g frozen blueberries

200ml coconut water

100ml water

200g kefir

½ teaspoon vanilla extract

½ teaspoon mixed spice

1 teaspoon maple syrup
   (optional)

1   Place all the
ingredients in a high-
powered blender and
blend to your desired
consistency.

_____ Tip _____

You can substitute any
dairy-free yoghurt into
this recipe, but it will likely
reduce the protein content.
You could add a scoop of
plant-based protein powder
to compensate.

NUTRITIONAL INFO PER SERVING

ENERGY 287 KCAL | FAT 7.9G | CARBS 38G | (OF WHICH SUGARS) 32G | PROTEIN 12G

ICED SPICED
GOLDEN
COCONUT LATTE

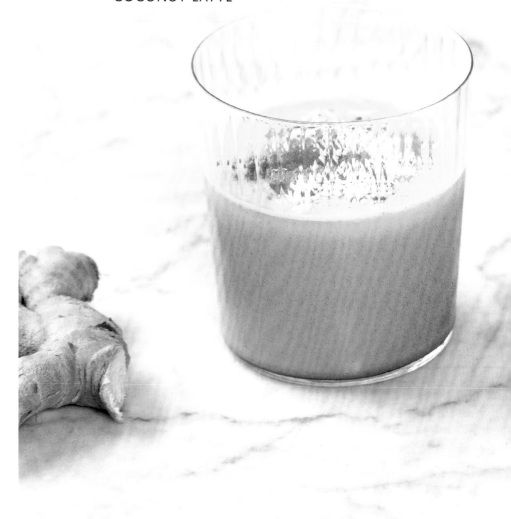

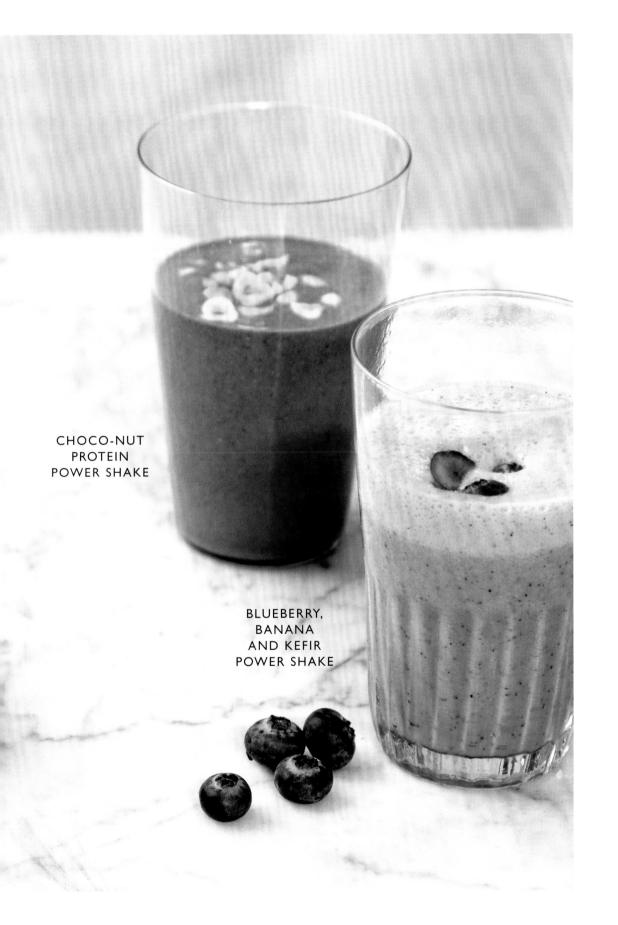

CHOCO-NUT
PROTEIN
POWER SHAKE

BLUEBERRY,
BANANA
AND KEFIR
POWER SHAKE

Blood orange, carrot and ginger juice

VEGAN | GLUTEN-FREE | DAIRY-FREE

___ *Tip* ___

SERVES 2

6 medium blood oranges
6 carrots
10cm piece of fresh root
    ginger, peeled

1 Halve and juice the oranges. Top and tail the carrots, scrub the skins and juice them with the skins on. Add the ginger to the juicer.

2 Mix well, chill, then serve.

For a cheat's version, use 250ml each of shop-bought carrot and blood orange juice. Or, if you want a drink with more fibre, blend the flesh of 2 large oranges and 2 carrots with the ginger in a high-powered blender.

NUTRITIONAL INFO PER SERVING

ENERGY 84 KCAL | FAT 0.5G | CARBS 17G | (OF WHICH SUGARS) 17G | PROTEIN 1.6G

Calming chamomile cooler

VEGETARIAN | GLUTEN-FREE | DAIRY-FREE

SERVES 2

1 chamomile tea bag
150ml freshly boiled water
1 teaspoon honey
1 mint leaf
couple of leaves of lemon
    thyme, or lemon verbena
200ml chilled apple juice
150ml chilled sparkling
    water

1 Steep a chamomile tea bag in the boiling water and leave to brew for 5 minutes. Stir in the honey, then set aside to cool to room temperature.

2 Finely chop the mint and lemon thyme or lemon verbena leaves. Combine with the cooled tea and leave to infuse at room temperature for 10 minutes, then chill.

3 Remove the tea bag. Strain to remove the herb leaves, if you like, add the chilled apple juice and sparkling water, then serve.

NUTRITIONAL INFO PER SERVING

ENERGY 46 KCAL | FAT 0G | CARBS 11G | (OF WHICH SUGARS) 10G | PROTEIN 0G

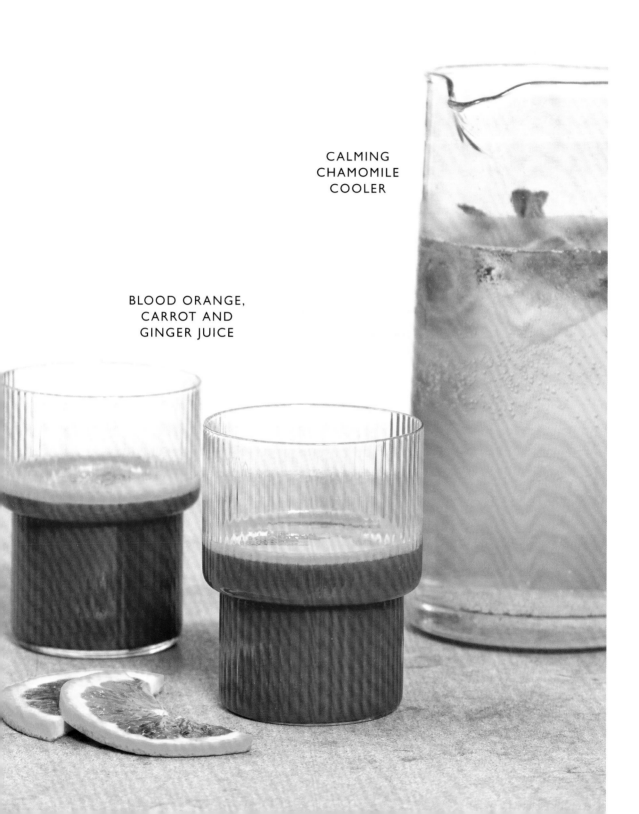

CALMING
CHAMOMILE
COOLER

BLOOD ORANGE,
CARROT AND
GINGER JUICE

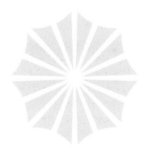

Dips & Salads

Edamame, mint and miso dip

VEGAN | GLUTEN-FREE | DAIRY-FREE

SERVES 4

120g frozen edamame
    beans, plus more
    (optional) to serve
leaves from 2 mint sprigs,
    plus more (optional)
    to serve
1 tablespoon olive oil
1 tablespoon miso paste
    (gluten-free)

finely grated zest and juice
    of ½ lemon, plus more
    zest (optional) to serve
sea salt (we use pink
    Himalayan) and freshly
    ground black pepper

1   Cook the edamame beans according to the packet instructions, then drain and leave to cool.

2   Place all the ingredients in a food processor and blend to your desired consistency. Serve scattered with lemon zest, mint leaves and edamame, if you like.

NUTRITIONAL INFO PER SERVING

ENERGY 78 KCAL | FAT 5.4G | CARBS 1.8G | (OF WHICH SUGARS) 0.8G | PROTEIN 4.5G

Sweet potato, smoked paprika and white bean dip

VEGAN | GLUTEN-FREE | DAIRY-FREE

SERVES 4

1 small sweet potato
    (around 150g), scrubbed
1 tablespoon olive oil, plus
    more to rub the potato
60g canned cannellini beans,
    drained weight, rinsed
1 garlic clove
1 teaspoon smoked paprika
sea salt and black pepper

1   Preheat the oven to 200°C (180°C fan), Gas Mark 6.

2   Rub the sweet potato with a little olive oil, season and bake for around 25 minutes, or until tender to the point of a knife. Scoop the flesh out into a bowl (or see tip, right) and leave it to cool.

3   Place the sweet potato flesh and all the other ingredients in a food processor and blend to your desired consistency.

_____ Tip _____

If you have a really powerful blender, you may be able to leave the skin on the sweet potato for extra fibre and still blend this dip to a smooth consistency.

NUTRITIONAL INFO PER SERVING

ENERGY 75 KCAL | FAT 3.4G | CARBS 8.8G | (OF WHICH SUGARS) 3.9G | PROTEIN 1.3G

Sun-dried tomato and lentil dip

VEGAN | GLUTEN-FREE | DAIRY-FREE

SERVES 4

120g cooked, cooled
   red lentils
80g sun-blush tomatoes,
   drained
1 teaspoon tahini
1 tablespoon water
20g rocket leaves
1 garlic clove

10g basil leaves, plus more
   (optional) to serve
juice of 1 lemon
sea salt (we use pink
   Himalayan) and freshly
   ground black pepper

1   Place all the
ingredients in a
food processor and
blend to your desired
consistency. Serve
scattered with a few
basil leaves, if you like.

_____ *Tip* _____

You can use other varieties
of lentil in this recipe if you
wish, but red lentils give it
a lovely colour. Green or
brown lentils can look a
little murky.

NUTRITIONAL INFO PER SERVING

ENERGY 97 KCAL | FAT 6.3G | CARBS 7.5G | (OF WHICH SUGARS) 2.9G | PROTEIN 3.8G

Champneys signature sweet and spicy bean dip

VEGAN | GLUTEN-FREE | DAIRY-FREE

SERVES 4

80g each canned kidney and
   mixed beans, drained
   weight, rinsed
¼ teaspoon chilli flakes,
   or to taste, plus more
   (optional) to serve
¼ teaspoon cumin seeds
1 tablespoon sweet chilli
   sauce (gluten-free)

1 tablespoon cold-pressed
   rapeseed oil
1 sun-dried tomato, drained
½ garlic clove
sea salt and freshly ground
   black pepper

1   Place all the ingredients in a food
processor and blend to your desired
consistency. Serve scattered with chilli
flakes, if you like.

NUTRITIONAL INFO PER SERVING

ENERGY 90 KCAL | FAT 4.5G | CARBS 7.7G | (OF WHICH SUGARS) 1.6G | PROTEIN 3.1G

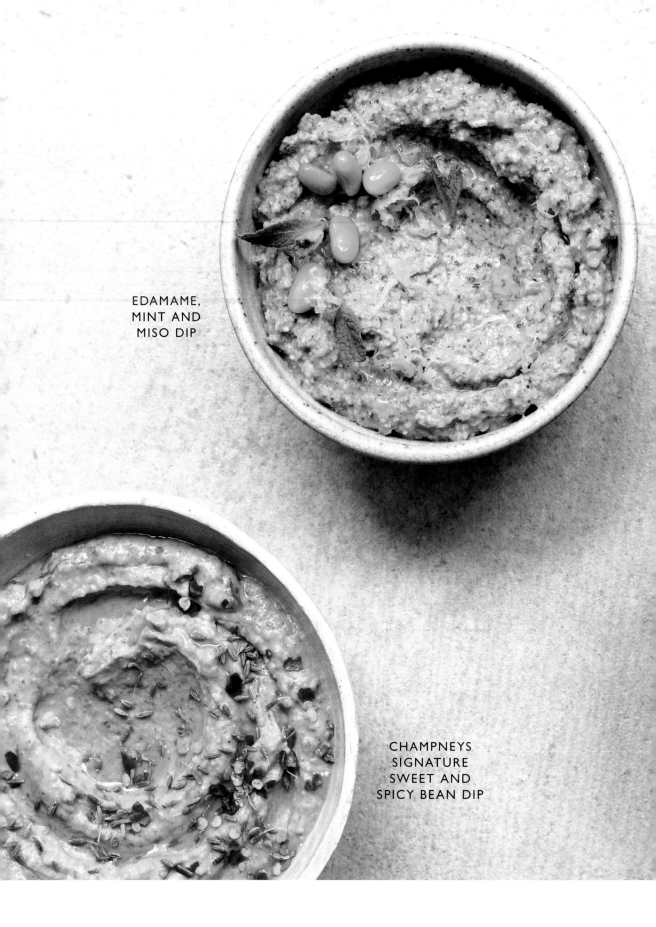

EDAMAME,
MINT AND
MISO DIP

CHAMPNEYS
SIGNATURE
SWEET AND
SPICY BEAN DIP

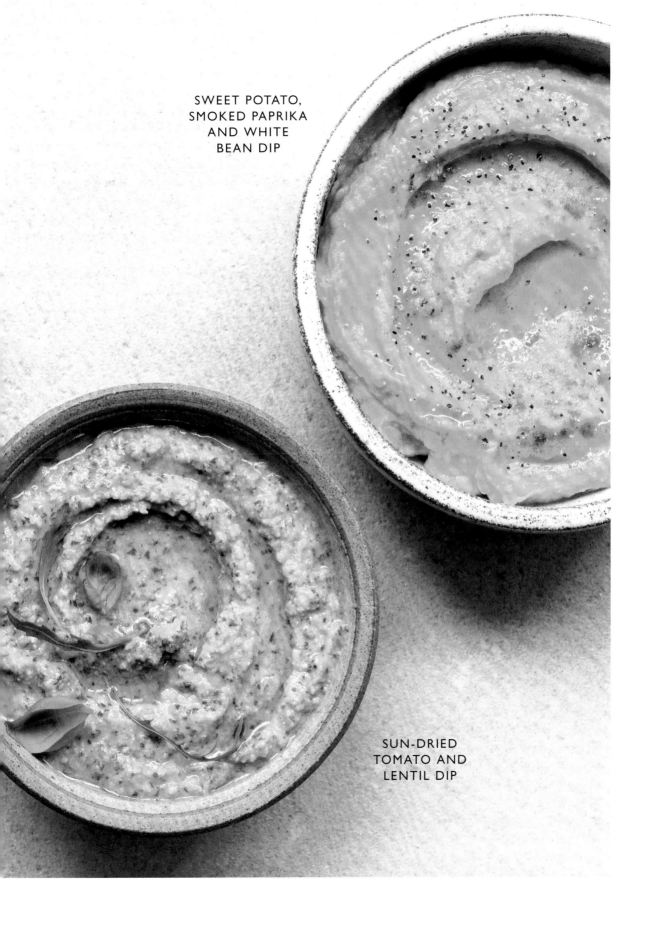

SWEET POTATO,
SMOKED PAPRIKA
AND WHITE
BEAN DIP

SUN-DRIED
TOMATO AND
LENTIL DIP

Green pea pesto dip

VEGAN | GLUTEN-FREE | DAIRY-FREE

SERVES 4

120g cooked, cooled peas

20ml olive oil

20g pine nuts

1 garlic clove

2 teaspoons lemon juice

2 basil sprigs

2 tarragon sprigs

leaves from 2 mint sprigs,
    plus more (optional)
    to serve

sea salt (we use pink
    Himalayan) and freshly
    ground black pepper

1 Place all the ingredients in a food processor and blend to your desired consistency. Serve topped with mint leaves, if you like.

Tip

Pine nuts can be pricey due to the time involved cultivating the nuts and the labour involved to extract pine nuts from pine cones. It can take a pine tree 50 years to reach prime pine nut producing stage! If you're looking for a more economical yet still tasty and healthy alternative try a 50:50 mix of pumpkin seeds and cashew nuts.

NUTRITIONAL INFO PER SERVING

ENERGY 112 KCAL | FAT 8.9G | CARBS 4G | (OF WHICH SUGARS) 2.1G | PROTEIN 2.7G

Beetroot and wasabi houmous

VEGAN | GLUTEN-FREE | DAIRY-FREE

SERVES 4

100g cooked beetroot
(about 1 large), natural
and not pickled

80g canned chickpeas,
drained weight, rinsed,
plus more (optional)
to serve

20g natural soya yoghurt
(gluten-free)

2 teaspoons olive oil

juice of ½ medium orange

1 teaspoon tahini

½ garlic clove

¼ teaspoon wasabi paste
(gluten-free)

sea salt (we use pink
Himalayan) and freshly
ground black pepper

1   Place all the ingredients in a food processor and blend to your desired consistency. Serve topped with chickpeas, if you like.

_____ *Tip* _____

This houmous looks and tastes beautiful on top of a baked sweet potato with some crumbled feta cheese and mint leaves.

NUTRITIONAL INFO PER SERVING

ENERGY 69 KCAL | FAT 3.7G | CARBS 5.6G | (OF WHICH SUGARS) 2.5G | PROTEIN 2.4G

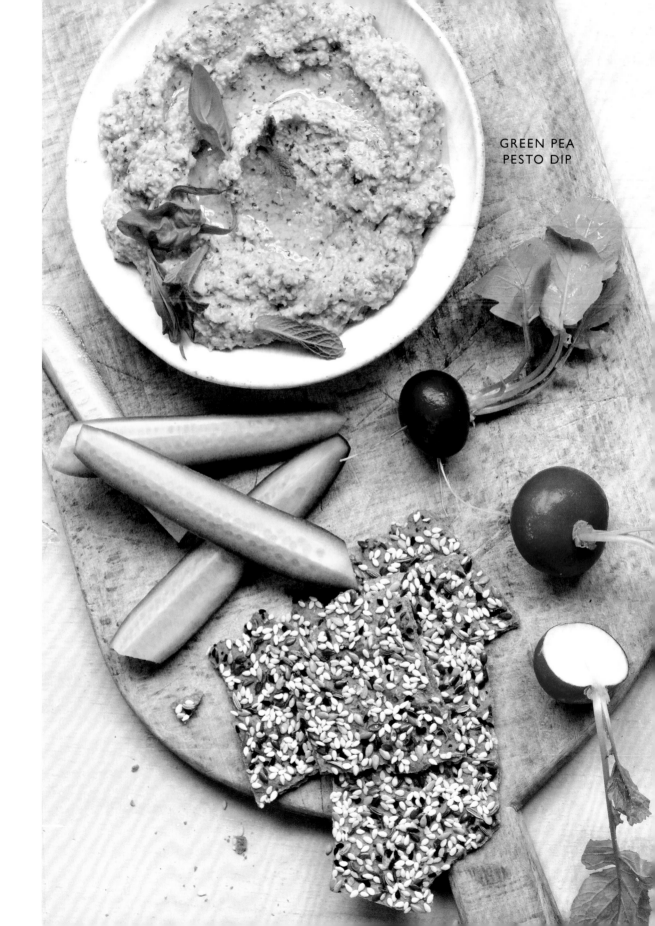

GREEN PEA
PESTO DIP

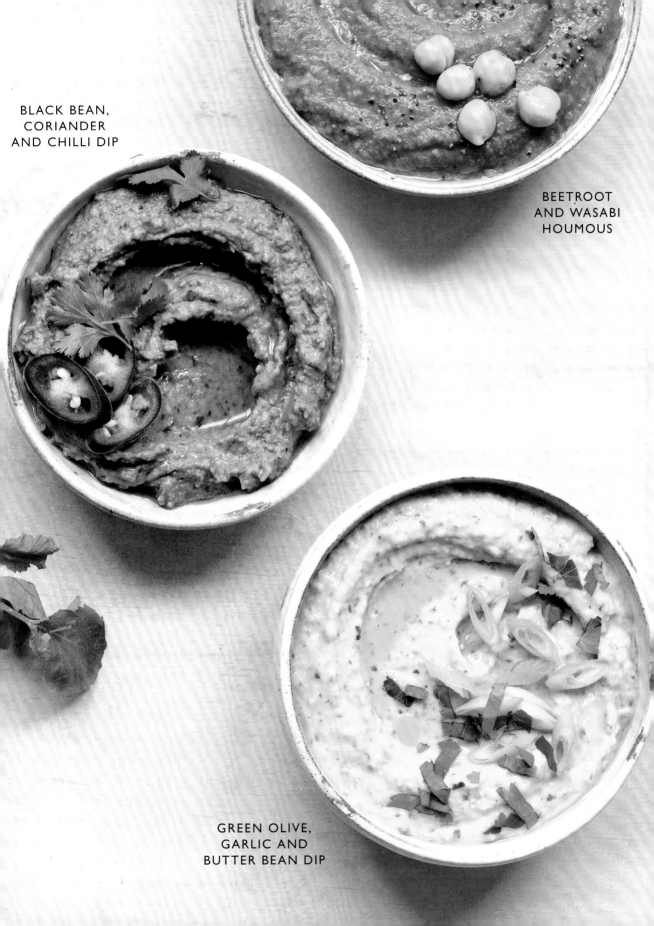

BLACK BEAN,
CORIANDER
AND CHILLI DIP

BEETROOT
AND WASABI
HOUMOUS

GREEN OLIVE,
GARLIC AND
BUTTER BEAN DIP

Black bean, coriander and chilli dip

SERVES 4

120g canned black beans, drained weight, rinsed

leaves from 2 coriander sprigs, or to taste, plus more (optional) to serve

1 tablespoon olive oil

1 tablespoon natural soya yoghurt (gluten-free)

1 garlic clove

½ green chilli, or to taste, plus more (optional) to serve

sea salt (we use pink Himalayan) and freshly ground black pepper

1 Place all the ingredients in a food processor and blend to your desired consistency. Serve scattered with chopped green chillies and coriander, if you like.

NUTRITIONAL INFO PER SERVING

ENERGY 67 KCAL | FAT 3.6G | CARBS 4.1G | (OF WHICH SUGARS) 1.7G | PROTEIN 3G

Green olive, garlic and butter bean dip

SERVES 4

120g canned butter beans,
    drained weight, rinsed

30g green olives

1 teaspoon tahini

2 tablespoons water

1 spring onion, plus more
    (optional) to serve

1 garlic clove

1 tablespoon natural
    soya yoghurt (gluten-free)

1 tablespoon olive oil

leaves from 2 parsley sprigs,
    plus more (optional)
    to serve

½ teaspoon dried oregano

squeeze of lemon juice

sea salt (we use pink
    Himalayan) and freshly
    ground black pepper

1   Place all the ingredients in a food processor and blend to your desired consistency. Serve scattered with chopped spring onions and parsley leaves, if you like.

Tip

Using beans and other pulses is a clever way to get more fibre and protein into your dips. They are also an easy ingredient to substitute, if you want to switch things up.

NUTRITIONAL INFO PER SERVING

ENERGY 71 KCAL | FAT 4.4G | CARBS 4.2G | (OF WHICH SUGARS) 0.7G | PROTEIN 2.5G

Champneys superfood salad

VEGAN | GLUTEN-FREE | DAIRY-FREE

SERVES 4

100g quinoa
60g frozen edamame beans
100g butternut squash
60g kale (weight of about
    ½ bunch after coarse
    ribs removed)
1 red pepper, sliced
80g cooked Puy lentils, from
    a pouch or can, drained
    and rinsed
30g pumpkin seeds
seeds of 1 pomegranate

FOR CHAMPNEYS
SIGNATURE DRESSING
4 tablespoons cold-pressed
    rapeseed oil
finely grated zest and juice
    of 1 lemon
1 tablespoon Dijon mustard
4 tablespoons chopped
    chives
3 tablespoons chopped
    parsley leaves
2 tablespoons chopped dill
sea salt (we use pink
    Himalayan) and freshly
    ground black pepper

1 Prepare the quinoa and edamame beans according to the packet instructions, then drain and cool.

2 Preheat the oven to 220°C (200°C fan), Gas Mark 7.

3 Peel and chop the squash into 2.5cm cubes and roast for around 20 minutes, or until tender to the point of a knife, then leave to cool.

4 Lightly steam the kale until softened – this should take 6–8 minutes – then transfer to iced water to stop the cooking process. Drain very well.

5 In a bowl, combine the quinoa, edamame, butternut squash, kale, red pepper and lentils.

6 Combine all the ingredients for the dressing in a separate bowl and whisk by hand, or blend in a food processor, until emulsified, seasoning well. Drizzle the dressing over the salad. Sprinkle with pumpkin and pomegranate seeds and serve.

Tip

A great hack for superfood kale is to massage the leaves with a little oil, salt and spices and bake them until crunchy. They can then take the place of potato crisps as a pre-dinner snack.

NUTRITIONAL INFO PER SERVING

ENERGY 341 KCAL | FAT 19G | CARBS 26G | (OF WHICH SUGARS) 8.9G | PROTEIN 12G

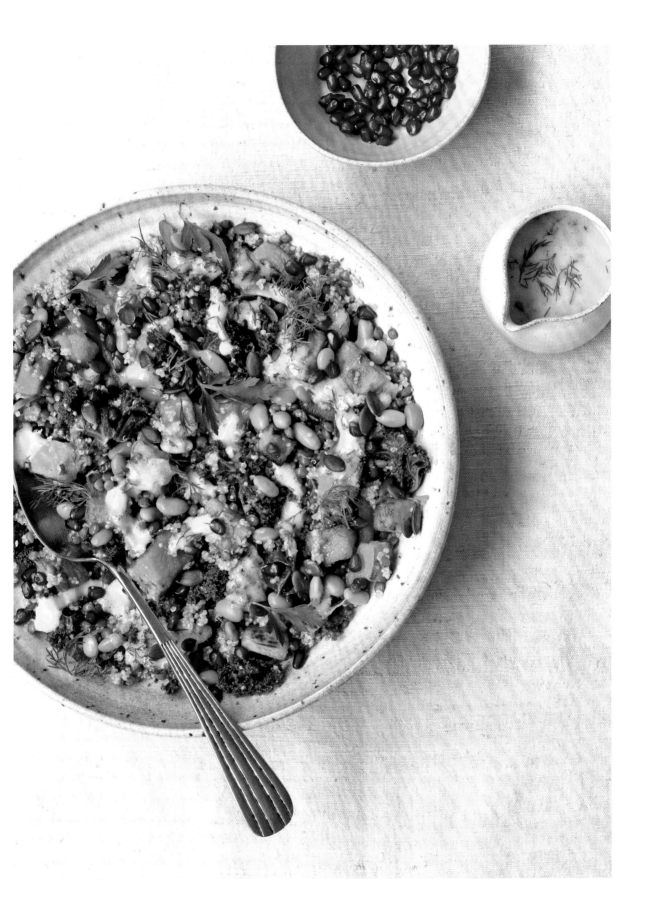

Clean green cucumber, avocado and caper salad

VEGAN | GLUTEN-FREE | DAIRY-FREE

SERVES 4

1 large cucumber, deseeded
   and sliced
1 ripe avocado, peeled,
   pitted and chopped
2 tablespoons capers,
   drained
1 tablespoon chopped
   coriander leaves
1 tablespoon chopped
   parsley leaves
1 tablespoon finely
   chopped chives
½ garlic clove, finely grated
   or minced
2 tablespoons olive oil
2 tablespoons lime juice
sea salt (we use pink
   Himalayan) and freshly
   ground black pepper

1 Put the cucumber in a large salad bowl with the avocado, capers, herbs and garlic. Sprinkle with salt and pepper to taste and drizzle with the olive oil and lime juice.

2 Toss gently to coat, then serve.

NUTRITIONAL INFO PER SERVING

ENERGY 170 KCAL | FAT 16G | CARBS 3.1G | (OF WHICH SUGARS) 2.3G | PROTEIN 2.6G

Rainbow ribbon slaw

with apple cider vinaigrette

VEGAN | GLUTEN-FREE | DAIRY-FREE

SERVES 4

1 large carrot
¼ medium red cabbage
2 large celery sticks
1 large green apple,
    skin on, cored
4 spring onions, finely sliced
40g walnuts, chopped

**FOR THE
VINAIGRETTE**
2 tablespoons olive oil
2 tablespoons apple
    cider vinegar
1 tablespoon wholegrain
    mustard
2 tablespoons water
sea salt (we use pink
    Himalayan) and freshly
    ground black pepper

1 Grate or shred the carrot, cabbage, celery and apple, using a food processor fitted with the shredder attachment, or on the coarse side of a box grater. Mix them with the spring onions and walnuts.

2 Combine all the ingredients for the vinaigrette dressing in a food processor and blend until smooth. Drizzle over the salad, toss gently to coat, then serve.

Tip

All sorts of raw vegetables can be ribboned into coleslaw. Try kohlrabi, or even broccoli stalks for a zero-waste approach.

NUTRITIONAL INFO PER SERVING

ENERGY 203 KCAL | FAT 14G | CARBS 13G | (OF WHICH SUGARS) 11G | PROTEIN 3.5G

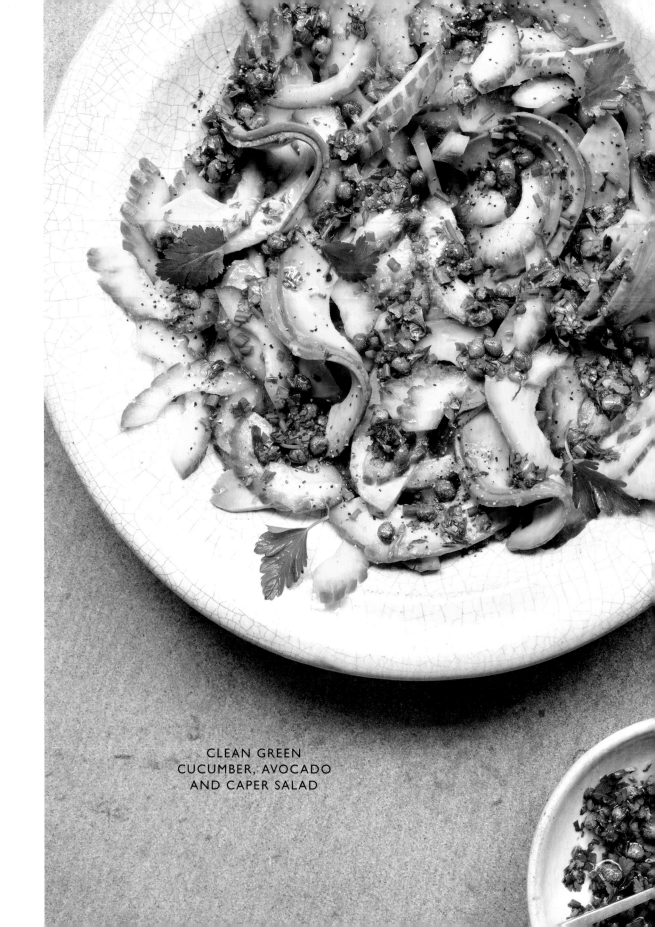

CLEAN GREEN
CUCUMBER, AVOCADO
AND CAPER SALAD

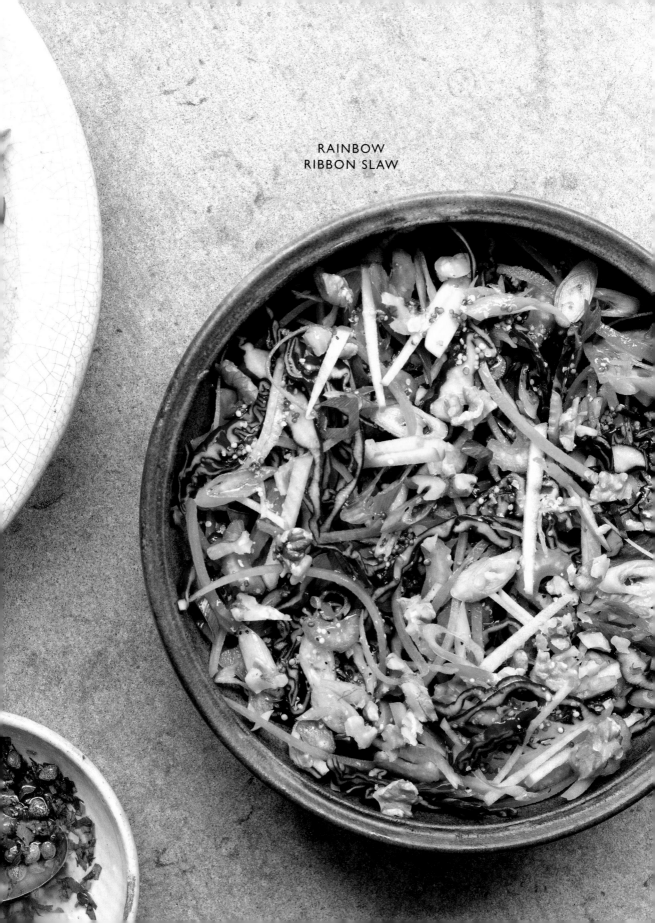

RAINBOW
RIBBON SLAW

Beetroot, apple and spinach salad
with hazelnuts and goat's cheese dressing

VEGETARIAN (DEPENDING ON THE GOAT'S CHEESE) | GLUTEN-FREE

SERVES 4

80g baby spinach

2 tablespoons chopped
parsley leaves

1 medium apple, skin on,
cored and finely sliced

1½ medium cooked
beetroots (120g),
roughly chopped

30g hazelnuts, halved or
roughly chopped

FOR THE DRESSING

40g soft goat's cheese

20ml semi-skimmed milk

1 tablespoon olive oil

2 tablespoons water

1 tablespoon honey

1 tablespoon white
wine vinegar

1   Put the spinach in a large bowl, then mix in the parsley leaves and apple. Arrange the beetroot pieces over the leaves.

2   Gently toast the hazelnuts in a dry frying pan for 2–3 minutes, then add them to the bowl.

3   Combine all the dressing ingredients in a food processor and blend until smooth and emulsified. Drizzle the dressing over the salad – but do not toss it – and serve immediately.

NUTRITIONAL INFO PER SERVING

ENERGY 177 KCAL | FAT 11G | CARBS 27G | (OF WHICH SUGARS) 12G | PROTEIN 5.1G

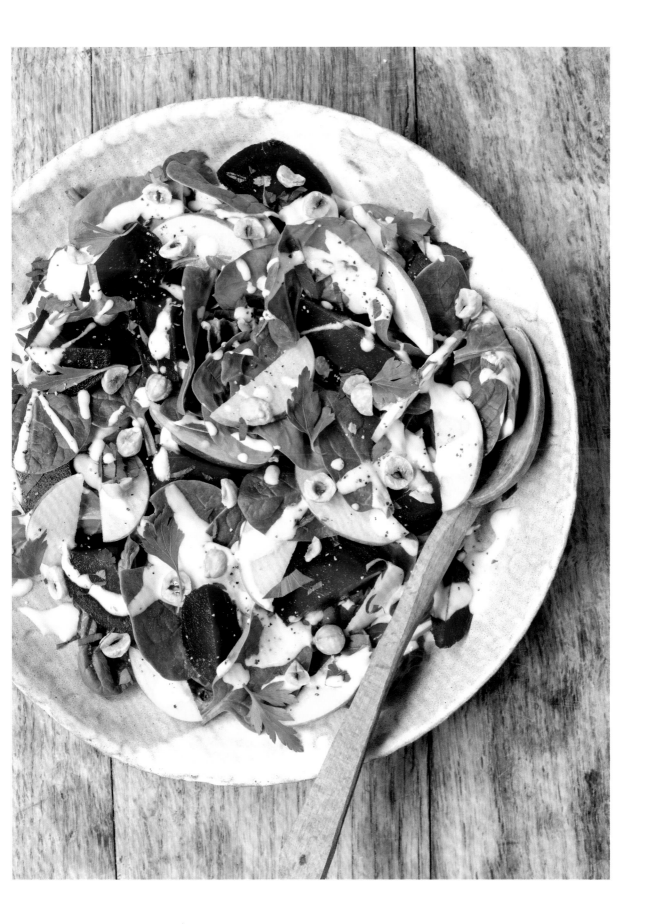

Celery, fennel and parsley salad
with sweet orange vinaigrette

VEGETARIAN | GLUTEN-FREE | DAIRY-FREE

SERVES 4

3 celery sticks (150g),
   finely sliced
½ fennel bulb (80g),
   finely sliced
20g parsley leaves, chopped

FOR THE VINAIGRETTE
finely grated zest and juice
   of ½ large orange
1 tablespoon cold-pressed
   rapeseed oil
1 tablespoon apple
   cider vinegar
1 tablespoon honey
½ garlic clove, finely grated
   or minced
pinch of sea salt (we use
   pink Himalayan salt)

1 Mix the celery, fennel and parsley in a bowl.

2 Put all the ingredients for the vinaigrette in a food processor and blend until emulsified. Drizzle over the salad and serve immediately.

Tip

Herbs are packed full of vitamins and minerals and should not be overlooked as a salad vegetable in their own right, rather than merely a garnish.

NUTRITIONAL INFO PER SERVING

ENERGY 115 KCAL | FAT 6.4G | CARBS 13G | (OF WHICH SUGARS) 11G | PROTEIN 0.9G

Coconut, coriander and lime cauliflower rice salad

VEGAN | GLUTEN-FREE | DAIRY-FREE

SERVES 4

80g wild rice
120g cauliflower florets
    (about ¼ cauliflower)
2 teaspoons olive oil
1 spring onion,
    finely sliced
2 tablespoons chopped
    coriander leaves
40ml canned coconut milk
15g desiccated coconut
finely grated zest and juice
    of ½ lime
sea salt (we use pink
    Himalayan) and freshly
    ground black pepper

1   Prepare the wild rice according to the packet instructions, then drain and set aside.

2   Place the cauliflower in a food processor with the olive oil and pulse-blend until it breaks down into rice-sized pieces. Do not let the food processor run, or you'll end up with white mush!

3   Heat a large frying pan and fry the cauliflower rice for 1–2 minutes, until warmed through. Add the wild rice, spring onion, coriander, coconut milk and desiccated coconut, salt and pepper. Mix well and warm through.

4   Once well combined, mix in the lime zest and juice and serve warm, or leave to cool, then serve.

NUTRITIONAL INFO PER SERVING

ENERGY 151 KCAL | FAT 7G | CARBS 16G | (OF WHICH SUGARS) 1.9G | PROTEIN 4.2G

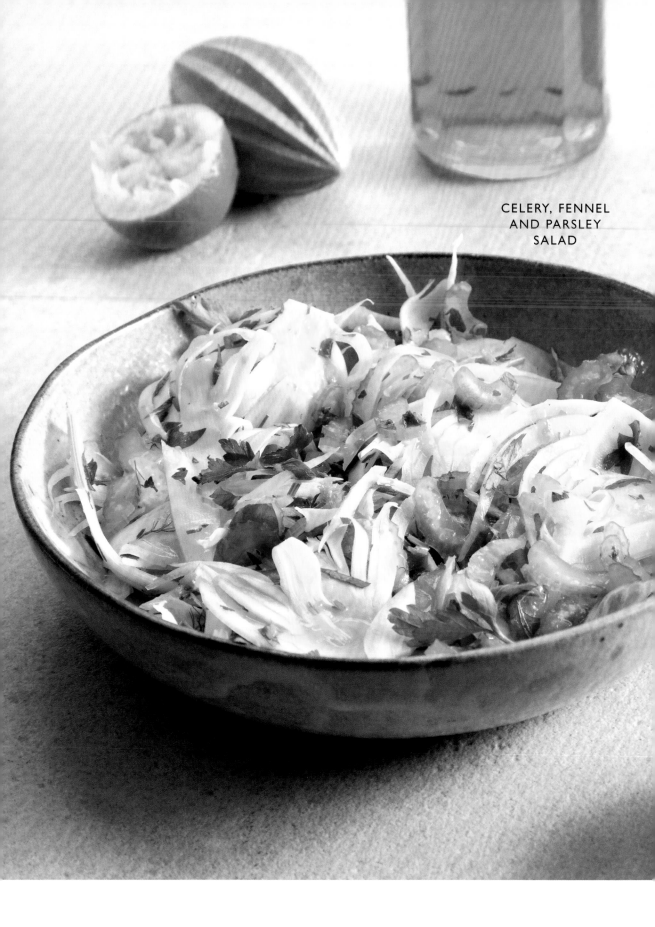

CELERY, FENNEL
AND PARSLEY
SALAD

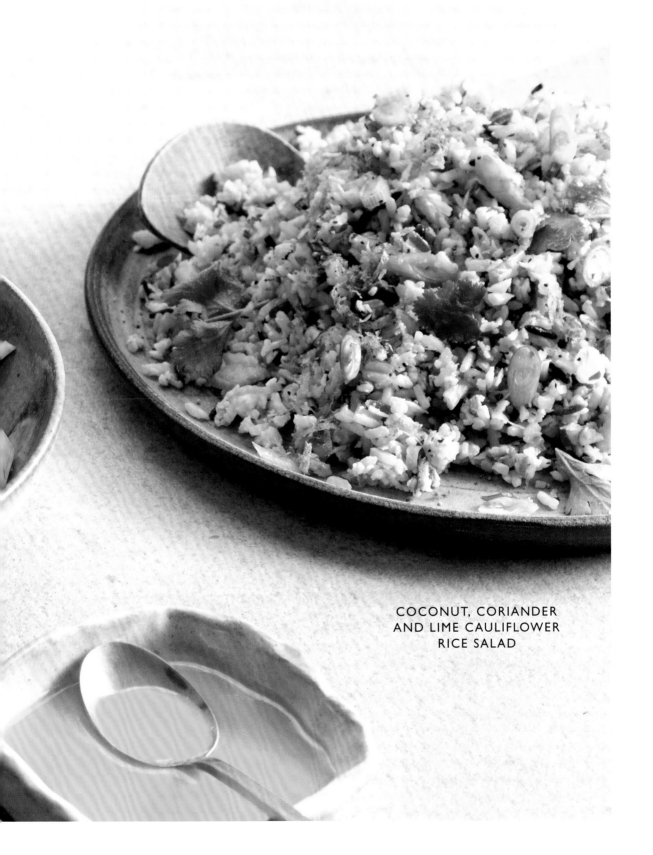

COCONUT, CORIANDER
AND LIME CAULIFLOWER
RICE SALAD

Sourdough panzanella
with tomato and fennel

VEGAN | DAIRY-FREE

SERVES 4

120g sourdough rye bread
with crust, ideally 1–2
days old, cut or torn
into chunks

4 tablespoons olive oil

40g roasted red pepper
from a jar, drained
weight, sliced

2 large tomatoes, deseeded
and cut into 2cm chunks

½ fennel bulb, tops
trimmed, bulb very
finely sliced

¼ red onion, finely sliced

25g black olives, pitted and
coarsely chopped

1 handful finely shredded
basil leaves

2 tablespoons balsamic
vinegar

sea salt (we use pink
Himalayan) and freshly
ground black pepper

1   Preheat the oven to 200°C (180°C fan), Gas Mark 6.

2   In a large bowl, toss the bread with half the olive oil.
Spread the bread out on a baking sheet and bake for
12 minutes, or until nicely toasted. Let cool, then return
to the bowl.

3   Add the roasted pepper to the croutons along with
the tomatoes, fennel, onion, olives and basil.

4   In a small bowl, whisk the vinegar with the
remaining olive oil. Season and pour over the salad.

5   Toss and let the panzanella stand for 5 minutes to
absorb all the flavours before serving.

NUTRITIONAL INFO PER SERVING

ENERGY 174 KCAL | FAT 9.3G | CARBS 17G | (OF WHICH SUGARS) 6.2G | PROTEIN 2.9G

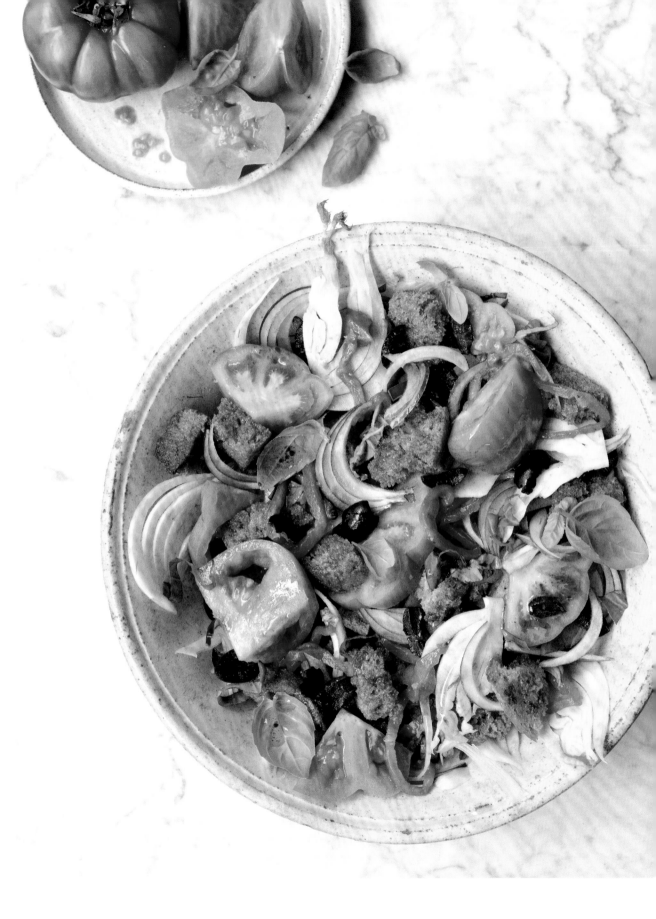

Shaved sprout, new potato and pumpkin seed salad
with maple-chilli dressing

VEGAN | GLUTEN-FREE | DAIRY-FREE

SERVES 4

150g new potatoes, boiled,
    cooled and sliced
100g Brussels sprouts,
    cored, peeled and
    finely shredded
½ red onion, finely sliced
20g dried cranberries
20g pumpkin seeds

FOR THE DRESSING
2 tablespoons olive oil
2 tablespoons sherry
    vinegar
1 tablespoon maple syrup
½ teaspoon chilli powder,
    or more if you like it hot!
2 tablespoons water
sea salt (we use pink
    Himalayan) and freshly
    ground black pepper

1   Toss the new potatoes, sprouts, red onion and cranberries together in a large bowl.

2   Dry-toast the pumpkin seeds in a frying pan for 2 minutes, then set aside to cool.

3   Put all the ingredients for the dressing in a mini food processor – or use a hand blender – and blend until smooth and emulsified, then season well. Add the dressing to the bowl of salad and toss well.

4   Sprinkle over the cooled pumpkin seeds to serve.

NUTRITIONAL INFO PER SERVING

ENERGY 155 KCAL | FAT 9.1G | CARBS 14G | (OF WHICH SUGARS) 7.2G | PROTEIN 3.3G

Griddled Baby Gem, butter bean and cauliflower salad

VEGAN | GLUTEN-FREE | DAIRY-FREE

SERVES 4

2 Baby Gem lettuces, cut
    into 8 wedges lengthways
2 tablespoons olive oil
½ medium cauliflower,
    trimmed and cut into
    small florets
1 teaspoon chopped
    rosemary leaves
1 tablespoon finely grated
    lemon zest, plus more
    to serve
1 tablespoon lemon juice
1 tablespoon red wine
    vinegar
80g canned butter beans,
    drained weight, rinsed
1 tablespoon chopped
    chives
1 tablespoon chopped
    parsley leaves
sea salt (we use pink
    Himalayan) and freshly
    ground black pepper
rocket leaves, to serve

1 Put the lettuces in a mixing bowl, drizzle with a little of the olive oil, then season.

2 Place a griddle pan over a high heat. Griddle the lettuce for 30–60 seconds on each side, or until slightly charred. Remove to a plate and allow to cool.

3 Steam the cauliflower florets for 5–6 minutes, or until al dente.

4 Combine half the remaining olive oil and the rosemary in a small saucepan. Stir over a medium heat just until fragrant (about 1 minute). Toss in the cauliflower for a further minute, then set aside to cool.

5 Whisk the lemon zest, juice and vinegar together in a small bowl and season well.

6 Combine the cauliflower, butter beans, lettuces, herbs and remaining oil in a bowl and toss. Season with salt and pepper and serve, sprinkling with lemon zest and rocket leaves.

NUTRITIONAL INFO PER SERVING

ENERGY 94 KCAL | FAT 6G | CARBS 5.5G | (OF WHICH SUGARS) 2.6G | PROTEIN 3G

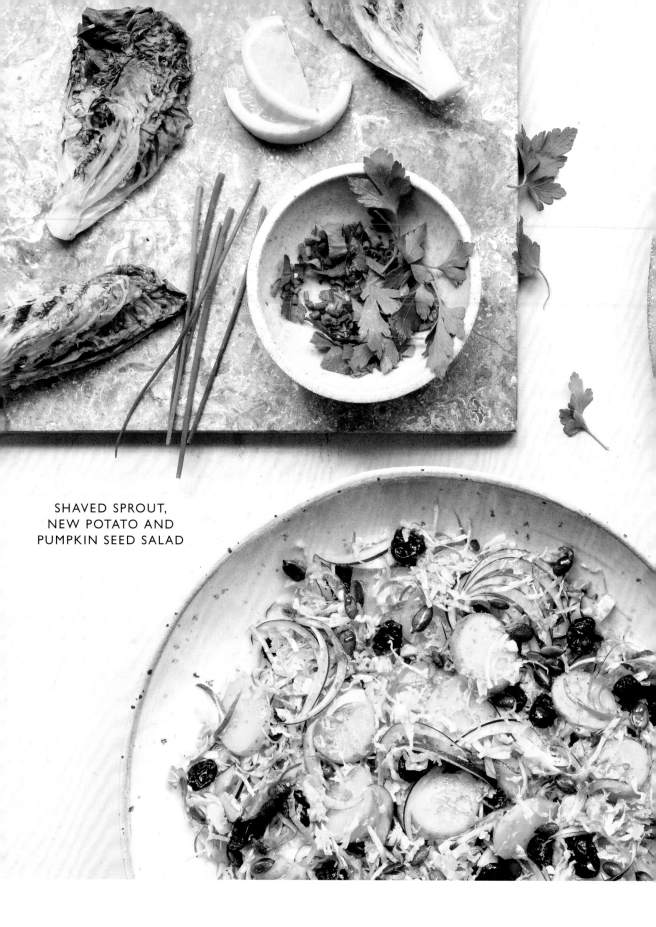

SHAVED SPROUT,
NEW POTATO AND
PUMPKIN SEED SALAD

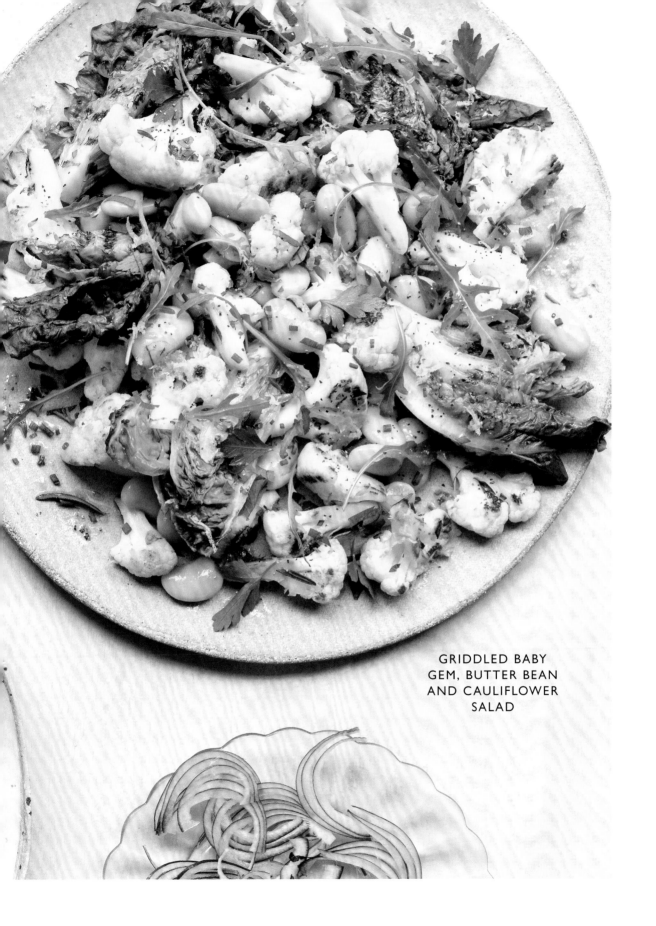

GRIDDLED BABY
GEM, BUTTER BEAN
AND CAULIFLOWER
SALAD

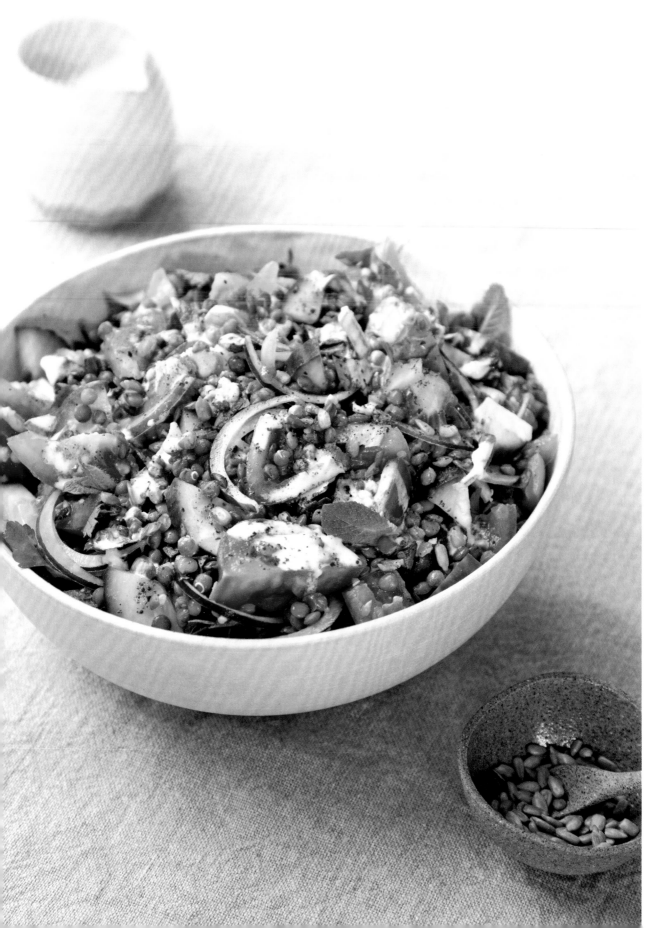

Puy tabbouleh
with creamy tahini–lemon dressing

VEGAN | GLUTEN-FREE | DAIRY-FREE

SERVES 4

200g cooked Puy lentils,
    drained weight, rinsed
2 medium tomatoes,
    chopped
½ red onion, finely sliced
¼ cucumber, chopped
20g mint leaves, chopped
20g parsley leaves, chopped
1 tablespoon sunflower
    seeds
½ teaspoon sumac
2 tablespoons olive oil

FOR THE DRESSING

45g natural soya yoghurt
    (gluten-free)
25g soya cream (gluten-free)
20g tahini
1 tablespoon cold-pressed
    rapeseed oil
2 tablespoons water,
    plus more (optional)
    if needed
1 garlic clove
finely grated zest and juice
    of 1 lemon, plus more
    juice (optional) if needed

1 Combine the lentils with the tomatoes, onion, cucumber, herbs, sunflower seeds and sumac. Dress with the olive oil and set aside.

2 For the dressing, combine all the ingredients in a food processor and blend well. Add a little more lemon juice or water if necessary to achieve a pourable dressing consistency.

3 Toss the tabbouleh in the dressing and serve.

NUTRITIONAL INFO PER SERVING

ENERGY 229 KCAL | FAT 15G | CARBS 12G | (OF WHICH SUGARS) 3.7G | PROTEIN 7.5G

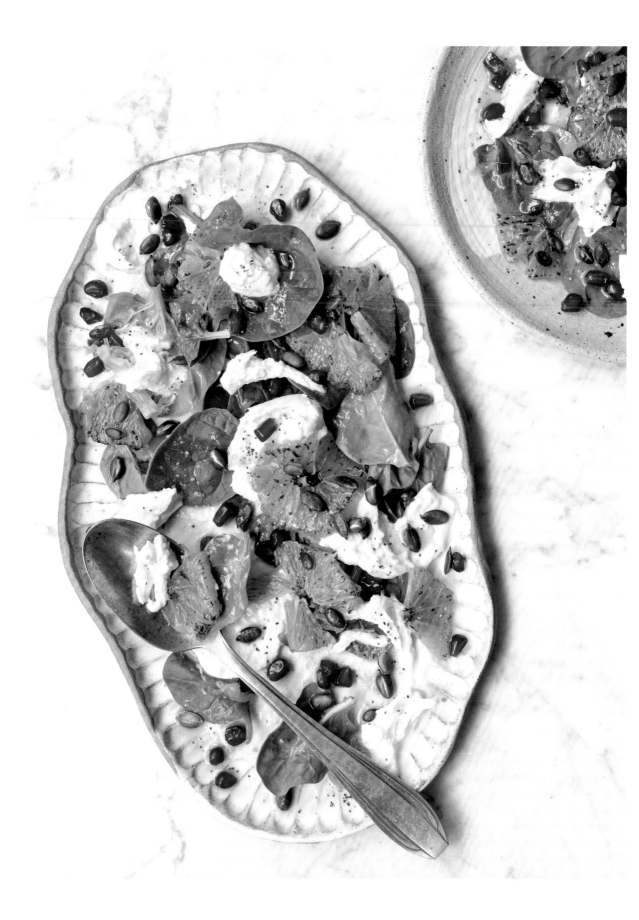

Spinach, mozzarella and caramelised pink grapefruit salad

GLUTEN-FREE

SERVES 4

1 pink grapefruit
40g pumpkin seeds
1 pomegranate
75g mozzarella, ideally
    buffalo mozzarella
100g baby spinach

FOR THE DRESSING
40ml flaxseed oil
1 teaspoon ground
    cardamom seeds
finely grated zest and juice
    of 1 lemon
sea salt (we use pink
    Himalayan) and freshly
    ground black pepper

1 Peel and segment the pink grapefruit. Grill or blowtorch the segments until caramelised.

2 Toast the pumpkin seeds for a couple of minutes in a dry frying pan, then set aside.

3 Remove the seeds from the pomegranate, keeping any juice for the dressing. Cut or tear the mozzarella and toss with the spinach and pomegranate seeds.

4 Whisk the flaxseed oil with any pomegranate juice you saved, the ground cardamom, lemon zest and juice and season to taste. Use this to dress the salad.

5 Serve the salad topped with the grapefruit segments and sprinkled with the toasted pumpkin seeds.

Tip

If you can get buffalo mozzarella rather than regular mozzarella, it gives this salad a really luxurious finish. Buffalo mozzarella is creamier, softer and more flavourful… but also a little more expensive!

NUTRITIONAL INFO PER SERVING

ENERGY 265 KCAL | FAT 19G | CARBS 12G | (OF WHICH SUGARS) 11G | PROTEIN 8.4G

Red rice and bean salad

*with avocado and mango, sesame,
lime and ginger dressing*

VEGAN | GLUTEN-FREE | DAIRY-FREE

SERVES 4

80g red rice
80g brown rice
200g canned mixed beans,
    drained weight, rinsed
½ large cucumber, chopped
2 large tomatoes, chopped
1 mango, peeled and
    chopped
80g rocket leaves
1 avocado, pitted
    and chopped
20g pumpkin seeds
2 tablespoons sesame
    seeds, toasted
1 teaspoon chilli flakes
2 spring onions, sliced

FOR THE DRESSING
2 teaspoons soy sauce
    (gluten-free), or tamari
finely grated zest and juice
    of 1 lime
2 tablespoons toasted
    sesame oil
5cm piece of root ginger,
    peeled and finely grated
sea salt (we use pink
    Himalayan) and freshly
    ground black pepper

1   Cook both types of rice according to the packet instructions, then drain and leave to cool.

2   Whisk together the dressing ingredients, or combine in a food processor, and blend until smooth and emulsified, seasoning well.

3   Place the rice in a large bowl with the beans, cucumber, tomatoes, mango, rocket and avocado. Pour over the dressing and toss, then season to taste.

4   Top with the pumpkin seeds, sesame seeds, chilli flakes and spring onions to serve.

Tip

If you can't find red rice (some shops only sell it as part of a mix), you can use wild rice in this salad instead, cooked according to the packet instructions.

NUTRITIONAL INFO PER SERVING

ENERGY 275 KCAL | FAT 12.3G | CARBS 36.6G | (OF WHICH SUGARS) 7.4G | PROTEIN 8.9G

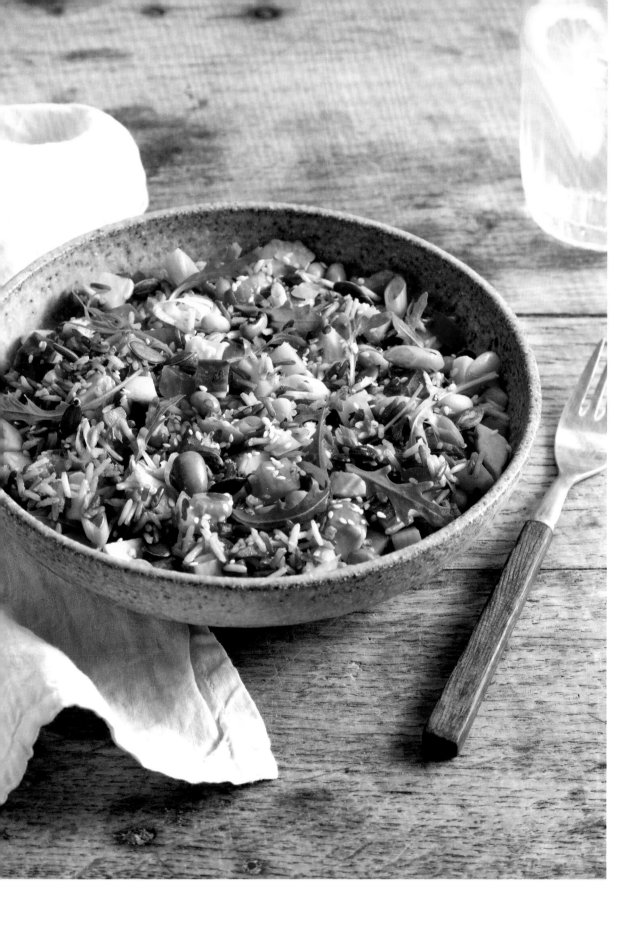

Avocado and kale salad
with pumpkin seed crunch, cashews and kimchi

GLUTEN-FREE | DAIRY-FREE

SERVES 2

200g kale (weight of
   about 2 bunches after
   coarse ribs removed),
   leaves chopped
1 teaspoon olive oil
2 garlic cloves, crushed or
   finely grated
10g sesame seeds
10g pumpkin seeds
10g sunflower seeds
10g raw cashews
10g root ginger, peeled
   and finely grated
2 teaspoons soy sauce
1 avocado
1 teaspoon wasabi paste
   (gluten-free)
finely grated zest and juice
   of 1 lime
200g kimchi (gluten-free)
sea salt (we use pink
   Himalayan) and freshly
   ground black pepper

FOR THE OPTIONAL
PROTEIN
EITHER
100g king prawns
OR
80g black beans, drained
   weight, rinsed
PLUS
olive oil spray
juice from the kimchi
   (see left)

1   In a sauté pan, cook the kale in the olive oil with the garlic, sesame seeds, salt and pepper for 3–4 minutes, until tender.

2   In a separate frying pan, dry-fry the pumpkin seeds, sunflower seeds and cashews with the ginger. Add the soy sauce.

3   If you're adding a protein, sauté the prawns or black beans in the same pan in which you cooked the kale, misting with olive oil spray, for 2–3 minutes. Add 1 tablespoon of juice from the kimchi for extra flavour.

4   Remove the stone from the avocado and scoop out the flesh. Roughly chop it and mash in a bowl with the wasabi, lime zest and juice, salt and pepper (or blend it, if you prefer a smooth consistency).

5   Arrange the kale, avocado, seeds and kimchi in 2 bowls or on 2 plates.

6   Serve the salad topped with your chosen protein, if you like.

___ Tip ___

Cooking elements of the
same recipe in one of the
pans already used for other
ingredients will add flavour
and consistency across
any dish.

NUTRITIONAL INFO PER SERVING (WITHOUT OPTIONAL PROTEIN)

ENERGY 312 KCAL | FAT 22.9G | CARBS 8.9G | (OF WHICH SUGARS) 3.3G | PROTEIN 9.8G

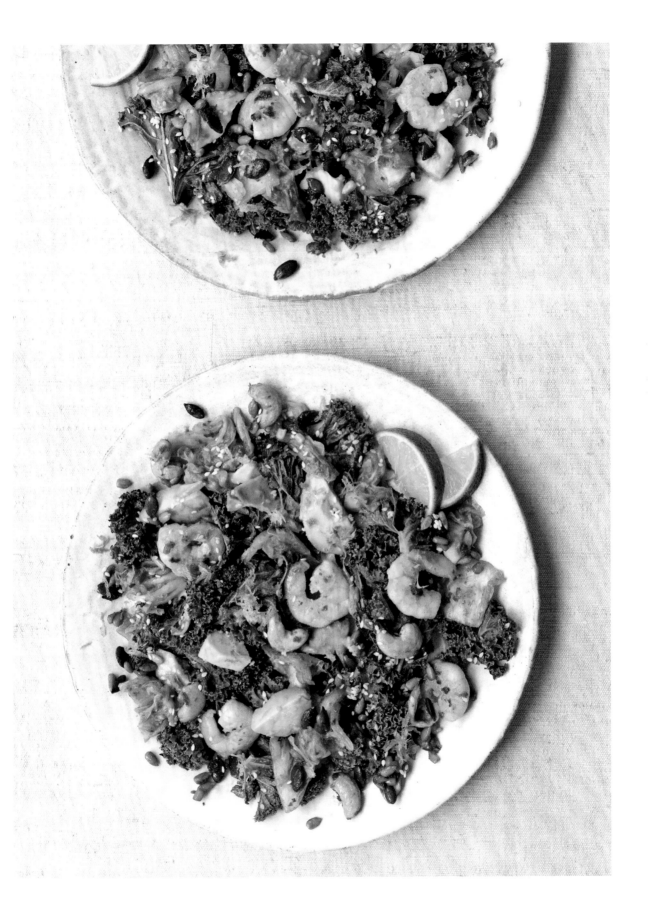

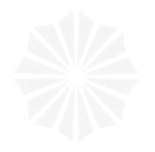

Lunch

Plant protein, pepper and paprika hash, sriracha sauce

VEGETARIAN | GLUTEN-FREE | DAIRY-FREE

SERVES 2

300g baby new potatoes, quartered

olive oil spray

1 garlic clove, crushed or finely grated

½ large onion, finely chopped

1 red pepper, finely chopped

1 teaspoon paprika

½ teaspoon chilli flakes

250g pulled plant-based 'meat' substitute (gluten-free)

2 spring onions, finely chopped

large handful of chives, chopped

large handful of coriander leaves, chopped

2 tablespoons sriracha sauce (gluten-free)

FOR THE OPTIONAL PROTEIN

EITHER

2 large eggs

1 teaspoon white wine vinegar

OR

60g mixed seeds

pinch each of smoked paprika, garlic salt (gluten-free) and cayenne pepper

1 Bring a large pan of water to the boil and cook the potatoes for 5 minutes, until slightly softened. Drain, then pat dry.

2 Heat a large frying pan and mist it with olive oil spray. Tip in the potatoes and cook for 10–15 minutes, until crisp on the outside and softened and fluffy on the inside.

3 Add the garlic, onion and pepper and cook for 5 minutes, or until softened but not coloured. Add the paprika and the chilli flakes and fry for 1 minute, until fragrant.

4 Meanwhile, prepare the pulled plant-based 'meat' substitute according to the packet instructions. Add it to the potatoes and cook until warmed through.

5 If you're adding eggs, crack each into a separate cup and bring a saucepan of water to the boil. Add the vinegar and reduce the heat to low. Stir the water to create a whirlpool and pour an egg into the vortex. Cook for 4–5 minutes, then lift out with a slotted spoon and drain while you cook the next egg.

6 If you're adding seeds, dry-fry them in a frying pan over a high heat for 2 minutes, adding the spices during cooking for extra flavour.

7 Scatter the spring onions, chives and coriander over the hash. Add your chosen protein, if using, then drizzle with sriracha sauce and serve.

NUTRITIONAL INFO PER SERVING (WITHOUT OPTIONAL PROTEIN)

ENERGY 280 KCAL | FAT 2.9G | CARBS 38.7G | (OF WHICH SUGARS) 9.3G | PROTEIN 21.9G

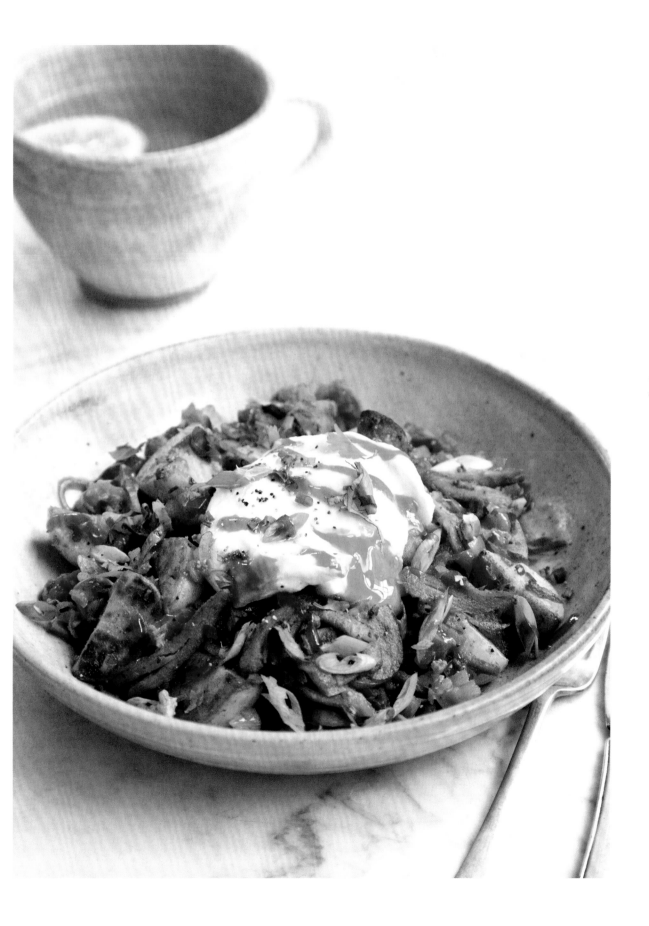

Protein-packed tomato, avocado, rocket and onion salad

VEGAN | GLUTEN-FREE | DAIRY-FREE

SERVES 2

100g firm tofu, sliced

½ teaspoon chilli flakes, plus more to serve

finely grated zest and juice of ½ lime, plus 2 tablespoons more lime juice for the avocado and to serve

200g large vine tomatoes

4 tablespoons balsamic vinegar

½ large onion, finely sliced

½ avocado

30g rocket leaves

2 handfuls of basil leaves

1 teaspoon olive oil

sea salt (we use pink Himalayan) and freshly ground black pepper

1   Grill or dry-fry the tofu slices until coloured; it should take 2–3 minutes on each side. Add the chilli flakes and lime juice to the pan to season and flavour during cooking.

2   Thickly slice the tomatoes, season with salt and pepper and dress with a little balsamic vinegar.

3   Arrange the tomato slices on a plate and add the sliced onion.

4   Slice the avocado chunkily and toss it with a little more lime juice. Add the chunky avocado slices to the tomato and onion and season everything well.

5   Place a few rocket leaves and most of the basil leaves over the avocado.

6   Top with the chunky tofu slices and sprinkle over more lime juice, the lime zest and a few extra chilli flakes and the remaining basil leaves to serve.

Tip

We've added citrus chilli tofu to this salad, though halloumi is delicious in its place, if you can eat dairy. Adding the protein of tofu or halloumi elevates this from a sassy side dish into a complete meal.

NUTRITIONAL INFO PER SERVING INCLUDING TOFU

ENERGY 210 KCAL | FAT 5.4G | CARBS 27.7G | (OF WHICH SUGARS) 15G | PROTEIN 17.8G

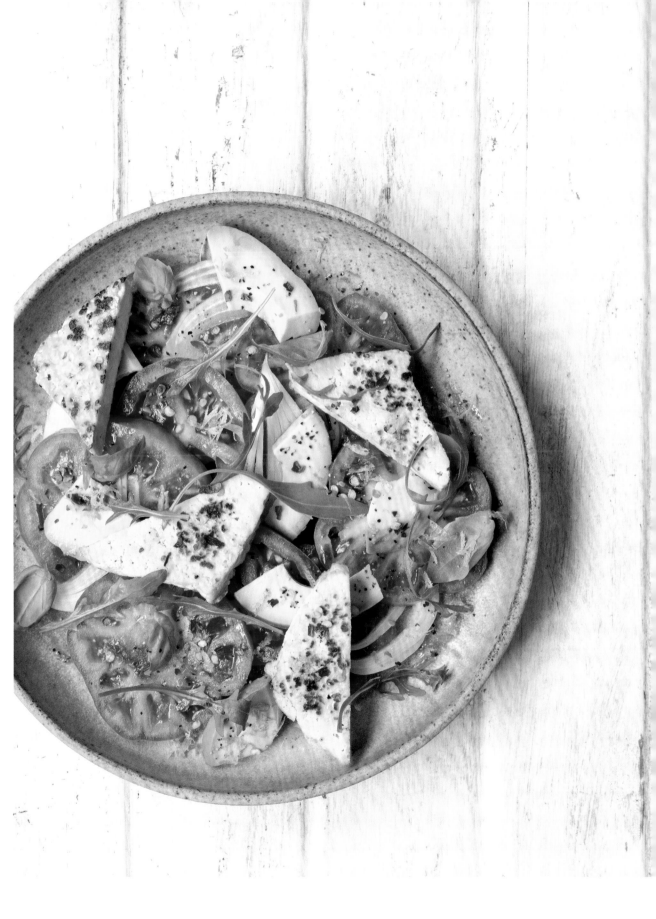

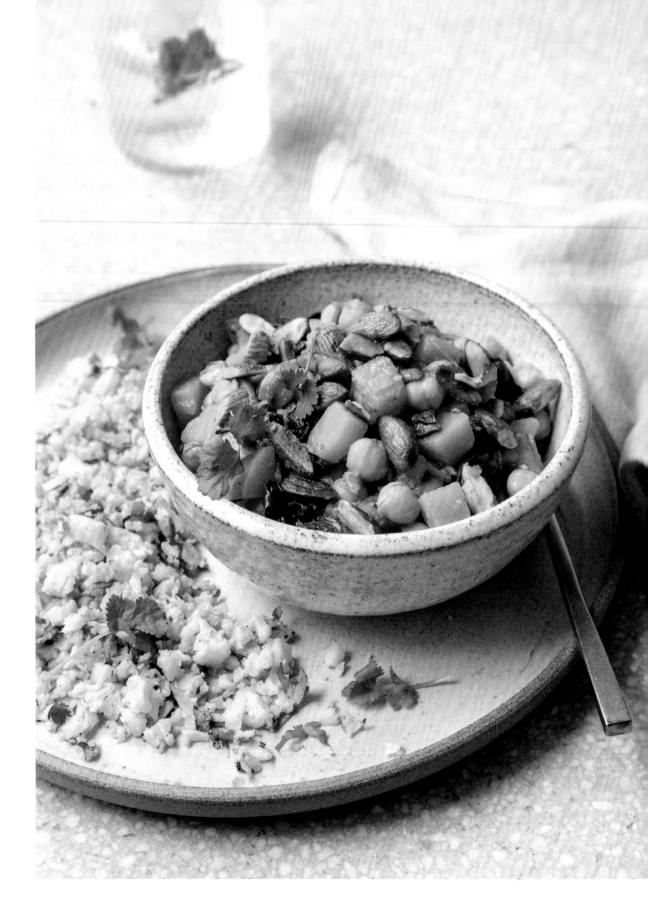

Butternut squash and chickpea curry, cauliflower rice

GLUTEN-FREE | DAIRY-FREE

SERVES 2

1 teaspoon coconut oil

½ large onion, chopped

2 garlic cloves, crushed
   or finely grated

5cm root ginger, peeled
   and finely grated

3 teaspoons curry paste
   (gluten-free)

½ teaspoon cinnamon

½ teaspoon coriander

½ teaspoon ground cumin

400g butternut squash,
   chopped

240g canned chickpeas,
   drained weight

200ml vegetable stock

50ml canned coconut milk

50g baby spinach

zest and juice of 1 lime

½ cauliflower, in florets

2 large handfuls of coriander

sea salt and black pepper

FOR THE OPTIONAL PROTEIN

EITHER

200g chicken breast

olive oil spray

OR

60g almonds, skin-on

¼ teaspoon curry powder
   (gluten-free)

1   Heat a large non-stick saucepan over a medium heat. Add the coconut oil and cook the onion, garlic and ginger for a couple of minutes until softened and starting to brown. Add 2 teaspoons of the curry paste if you're adding chicken later, otherwise add all 3 teaspoons. Add the cinnamon, ground coriander and cumin with a splash of water and cook for another minute.

2   Mix in the butternut squash and chickpeas to coat in the spices, then add the stock and coconut milk, season and bring to the boil. Cover and simmer for 15–20 minutes until the squash is tender, then add the spinach and lime juice (reserve the zest) and cook for a final couple of minutes.

3   If you're adding chicken, chop it into 2.5cm cubes and separately sauté them in olive oil spray with the remaining 1 teaspoon curry paste until cooked through, with slightly browned edges.

4   If you're adding almonds, dry-fry them in a frying pan over a high heat for 2–3 minutes until toasted. Toss in a little salt and pepper along with the ¼ teaspoon curry powder.

5   Place the cauliflower in a food processor and pulse-blend until it breaks down into rice-sized pieces. Do not let the food processor run, or you'll end up with white mush.

6   Sauté the cauliflower rice in olive oil spray in a sauté pan for 4–5 minutes until cooked with just a little colour, adding seasoning, the lime zest and half the coriander.

7   Add your chosen protein to the curry, if using.

8   Serve the curry with the cauliflower rice and sprinkle with the remaining chopped coriander.

NUTRITIONAL INFO PER SERVING (WITHOUT OPTIONAL PROTEIN)

ENERGY 274 KCAL | FAT 9.1G | CARBS 36.1G | (OF WHICH SUGARS) 8.2G | PROTEIN 15.4.G

Thai vegetable broth
with smoked tofu

GLUTEN-FREE | DAIRY-FREE

SERVES 2

1 medium-large carrot

150g chunk of mooli

1 teaspoon coconut oil (we use raw organic extra-virgin)

160g firm smoked tofu, cut into cubes

2 garlic cloves, crushed or finely grated

5cm piece of root ginger, peeled and finely grated

½ red chilli, finely sliced, or to taste

1 head of pak choi, quartered

1 red pepper, finely sliced

1.1 litres vegetable stock (gluten-free)

dash of tamari sauce

finely grated zest and juice of ½ lemon

large handful of coriander, chopped

large handful of mint leaves, chopped

sea salt (we use pink Himalayan) and freshly ground black pepper

100g brown rice, cooked, to serve

FOR THE OPTIONAL PROTEIN
EITHER
160g salmon fillet
OR
150g frozen edamame beans, defrosted
PLUS
olive oil spray
squeeze of lemon juice

1   Peel the carrot and mooli and ribbon them with a vegetable peeler or mandolin.

2   Heat a large saucepan with the coconut oil and sauté the tofu with the garlic, ginger and chilli until it has some colour (4–5 minutes). Add the ribboned carrot and mooli, the pak choi and pepper and cook through for a couple of minutes.

3   Combine the vegetable stock in a jug with the tamari, lemon zest and juice and pour this over the vegetable mixture. Bring to the boil, then reduce the heat to a simmer and cook for a few minutes until the liquid has reduced by half.

4   Meanwhile, cook the protein, if using. If you are cooking salmon, preheat the oven to 200˚C (180˚C fan), Gas Mark 6. For either salmon or edamame beans, heat a frying pan over a high heat and mist it with olive oil spray. Place the salmon in the pan – skin side down – or the beans and cook for 3 minutes (the fish skin, if using, should be crispy). Add salt, pepper and the lemon juice. The edamame are now ready. Transfer the salmon to the oven for 6–7 minutes until cooked through.

5   Serve the tofu and vegetables on a bed of the brown rice with the salmon or edamame, if using, then pour over the liquid from the pan. Scatter with the chopped coriander and mint, then serve.

NUTRITIONAL INFO PER SERVING (WITHOUT OPTIONAL PROTEIN)

ENERGY 302 KCAL | FAT 3.9G | CARBS 57G | (OF WHICH SUGARS) 12.2G | PROTEIN 12.9G

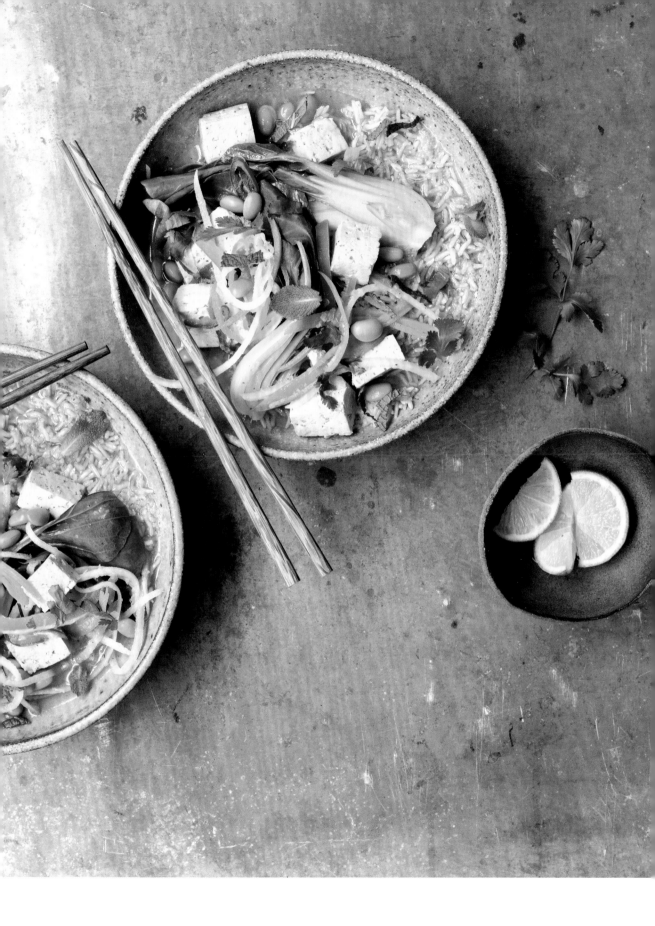

Maple-glazed salmon, samphire, Savoy cabbage, sauce vierge

GLUTEN-FREE | DAIRY-FREE

SERVES 2

100g plum tomatoes

10g basil leaves, finely sliced

10g coriander leaves, finely sliced

10g parsley leaves, finely sliced

juice of 1 lemon, plus lemon wedges to serve

2 medium salmon fillets

2 teaspoons maple syrup

½ Savoy cabbage, shredded

50g samphire

2 teaspoons olive oil

sea salt (we use pink Himalayan) and freshly ground black pepper

1 Preheat the oven to 200°C (180°C fan), Gas Mark 6.

2 Score each tomato on the base with a sharp knife, place in a large heatproof bowl and pour over just-boiled water from a kettle. After 15–30 seconds, you should be able to peel off the skins as they come away from the score marks. Cut into quarters and remove the pips and juice, then finely chop the flesh.

3 Mix the chopped tomatoes with the herbs and lemon juice and season well. Set this sauce vierge aside.

4 Put the salmon fillets on a baking tray, brush them with the maple syrup and bake for 6 minutes.

5 Meanwhile, bring 2 pans of lightly salted water to the boil. Blanch the cabbage for 1 minute and the samphire separately for 5 seconds. Drain both, then toss the cabbage with the olive oil.

6 Place the dressed cabbage on 2 plates, then add the fish fillets and top with the samphire. Pour over the sauce and serve with lemon wedges.

NUTRITIONAL INFO PER SERVING

ENERGY 290 KCAL | FAT 11.5G | CARBS 10.8G | (OF WHICH SUGARS) 7.8G | PROTEIN 36.6G

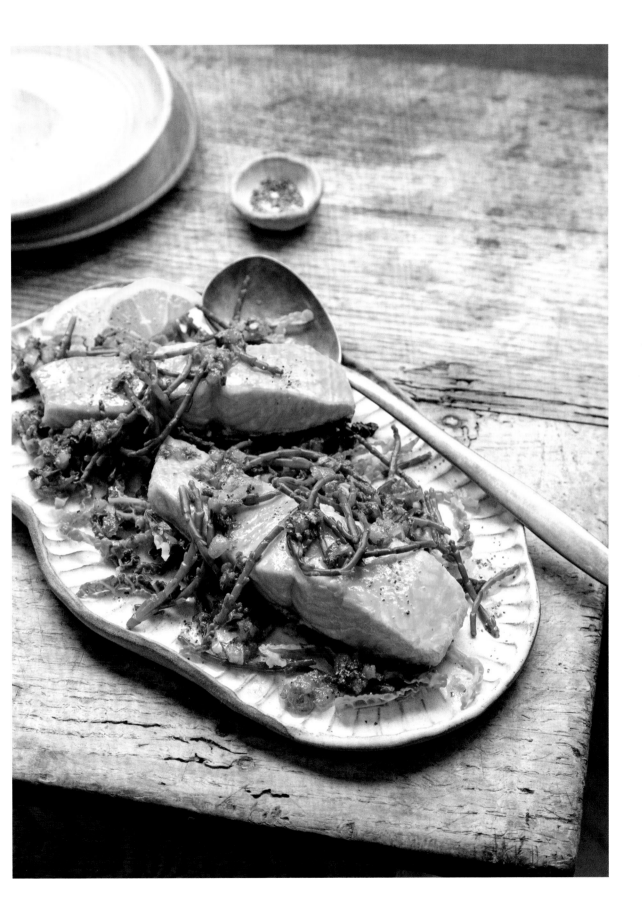

Roasted sea bass, aubergine caviar and corn salsa

GLUTEN-FREE | DAIRY-FREE

SERVES 2

FOR THE AUBERGINE
1 aubergine
1 garlic clove
1 teaspoon thyme leaves
2 teaspoons olive oil

FOR THE CORN SALSA
1 tablespoon vegetable oil
1 large shallot, very
    finely chopped
1 garlic clove, finely grated
½ red pepper, very
    finely chopped
½ yellow pepper, very
    finely chopped
100g sweetcorn
a little olive oil
juice of 1 lemon
100g cherry tomatoes,
    quartered
10g coriander leaves,
    finely chopped
10g basil leaves, finely
    chopped
10g chives, finely chopped
sea salt (we use pink
    Himalayan) and freshly
    ground black pepper

2 large sea bass fillets

1   Preheat the oven to 200°C (180°C fan), Gas Mark 6.

2   Make small holes with a fork in the aubergine. Place on a baking tray and cook for 45–60 minutes, or until dark and soft all the way through, turning frequently. When cooked, remove as much of the skin as possible. At the same time, wrap the garlic and thyme in a twist of foil and bake for 10–12 minutes until soft, then remove.

3   Put the cooked garlic and aubergine into a blender and blend, adding a little olive oil at a time to create the desired consistency. Season and pass through a sieve, if you want a very fine texture.

4   For the salsa, heat the vegetable oil in a heavy-based saucepan and sauté the shallot, garlic and peppers for a couple of minutes, seasoning well. Add the sweetcorn and just enough olive oil to bind, then finish with the lemon juice, cherry tomatoes and herbs, seasoning well.

5   Place the sea bass fillets on a baking tray and roast in the oven for 5–7 minutes. Leave to rest for 2 minutes.

6   Swipe the aubergine caviar over 2 plates and add the sea bass and corn salsa to serve.

NUTRITIONAL INFO PER SERVING

ENERGY 374 KCAL | FAT 22.1G | CARBS 10.2G | (OF WHICH SUGARS) 5.9G | PROTEIN 32.2G

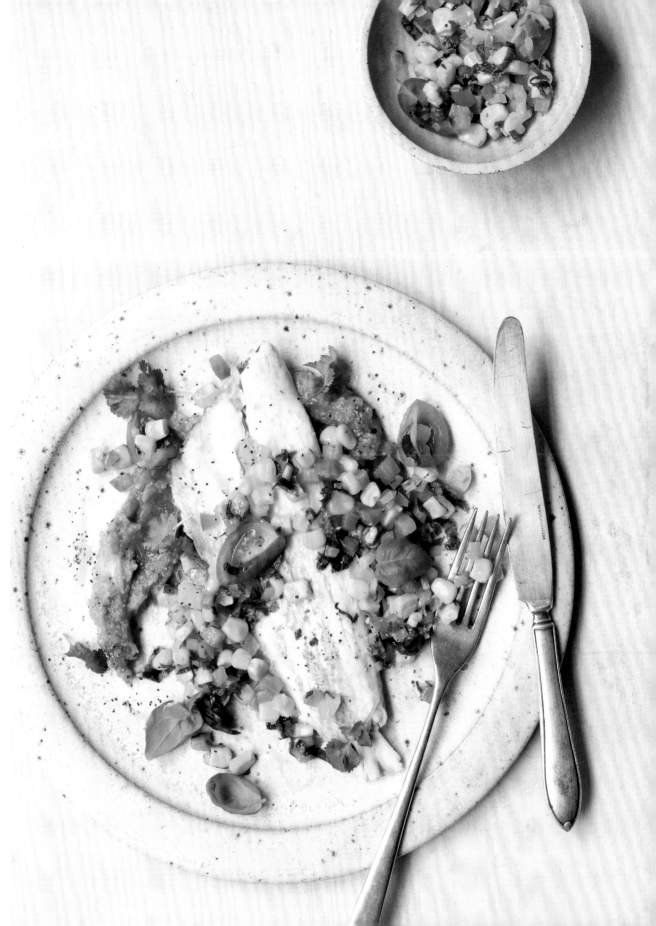

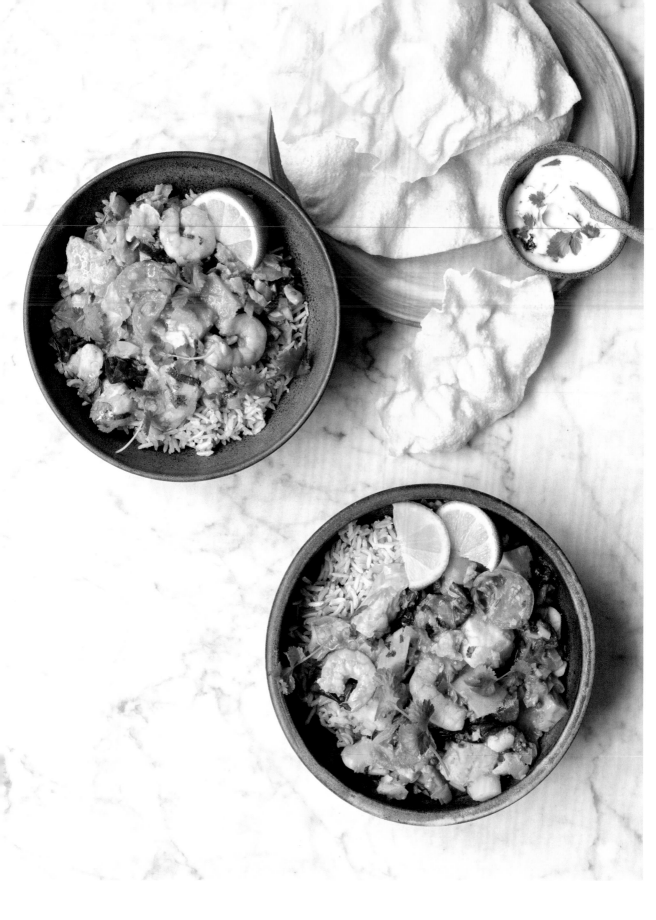

Seafood and sweet potato tikka masala

GLUTEN-FREE | DAIRY-FREE

SERVES 2

FOR THE SAUCE
½ teaspoon coriander seeds
2 garlic cloves, chopped
5g root ginger, peeled and
    roughly chopped
3 cardamom pods
I teaspoon curry powder
    (gluten-free)
½ teaspoon paprika
2 tablespoons tomato purée
½ teaspoon cumin seeds
finely grated zest and juice
    of ½ lemon
I shallot, roughly chopped
3 tablespoons water

FOR THE CURRY
I teaspoon coconut oil
    (we use raw organic
    extra-virgin)
I onion, finely chopped
½ small leek, finely chopped
3 large garlic cloves, crushed
    or finely grated
20g root ginger, peeled and
    finely grated
200g sweet potato, peeled
    and chopped
100g cherry tomatoes,
    chopped
100ml canned coconut milk

50ml water
200g mixed seafood,
    defrosted if frozen
50g baby spinach, defrosted
    if frozen
20g coriander leaves,
    chopped
finely grated zest and juice
    of ½ lime

TO SERVE (OPTIONAL)
100g brown rice
natural dairy-free yoghurt
2 plain poppadoms
    (gluten-free)
lime wedges

1 Combine all the tikka masala sauce ingredients in a food processor and blend until smooth.

2 Heat the coconut oil in a large sauté pan and cook the onion, leek, garlic and ginger until softened, but not coloured. Add the sweet potato, cherry tomatoes, coconut milk and measured water. Bring to the boil, then reduce the heat to a simmer and cook until the sweet potato is soft.

3 Add the mixed seafood and the tikka masala sauce, stirring it in gently. Add the spinach and most of the coriander and simmer for 5–10 minutes, until the sauce has reduced a little. Taste and adjust the acidity with the lime zest and juice.

4 Serve the curry on a bed of brown rice with yoghurt, poppadoms and lime wedges on the side, if you like, scattered with the remaining coriander.

NUTRITIONAL INFO PER SERVING

ENERGY 682 KCAL | FAT 12.7G | CARBS 121.3G | (OF WHICH SUGARS) 11.3G | PROTEIN 28.1G

Peri peri chicken leg, tamarind-coconut beans

SERVES 2

2 skin-on chicken legs
2 teaspoons peri peri
    seasoning (gluten-free)
½ teaspoon mixed spice
leaves from 2 thyme sprigs,
    finely chopped
leaves from 1 rosemary
    sprig, finely chopped
2 teaspoons olive oil
1 large shallot, finely
    chopped
1 garlic clove, crushed or
    finely chopped
2 teaspoons peeled and
    finely grated root ginger
1 red or yellow pepper,
    finely chopped
100ml vegetable stock
    (gluten-free)
2 teaspoons tamarind paste
200ml canned coconut milk
100g canned butter beans,
    drained weight, rinsed

10g coriander leaves, finely
    chopped, plus more
    to serve
leaves from 2 tarragon
    sprigs, finely chopped,
    plus more to serve
sea salt (we use pink
    Himalayan) and freshly
    ground black pepper
green vegetables, to serve

1   Score the skin of the chicken legs lightly on each side, then place in a dish and rub them with the peri peri seasoning and mixed spice, thyme and rosemary. Cover and refrigerate overnight.

2   The next day, preheat the oven to 200°C (180°C fan), Gas Mark 6.

3   Put the chicken legs on a baking tray and bake for 35 minutes, then remove from the oven and leave to rest for 5 minutes.

4   Heat the oil in a sauté pan and cook the shallot, garlic, ginger and pepper; they should soften but not colour. Pour in the stock and allow it to reduce by half. Add the tamarind paste and coconut milk and simmer for a few minutes.

5   Add the butter beans and reduce again until the sauce has the consistency of single cream, then season and finish with the coriander and tarragon.

6   Serve the chicken legs on the beans, sprinkled with herbs, with green vegetables on the side.

NUTRITIONAL INFO PER SERVING

ENERGY 395 KCAL | FAT 24.8G | CARBS 17.6G | (OF WHICH SUGARS) 4.6G | PROTEIN 32G

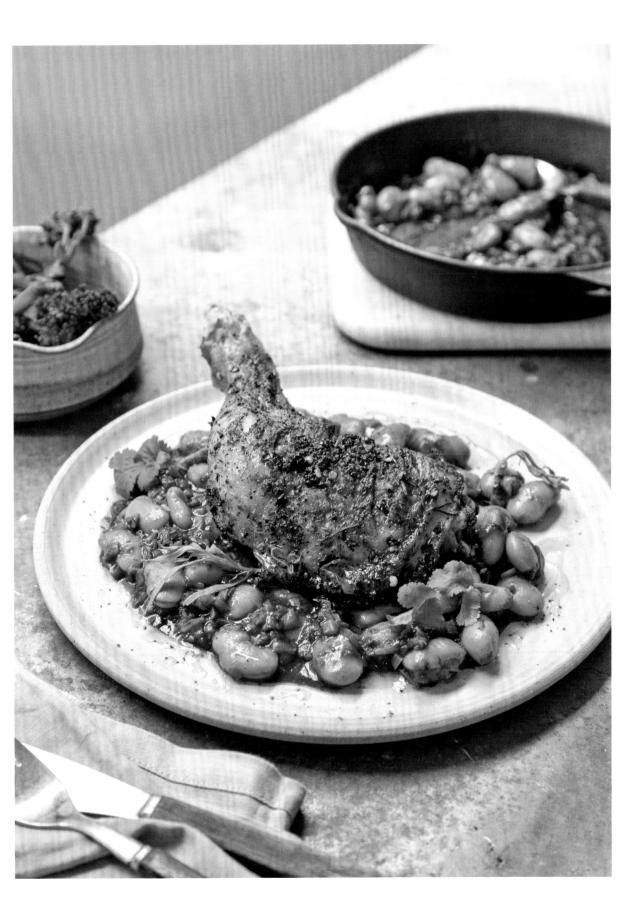

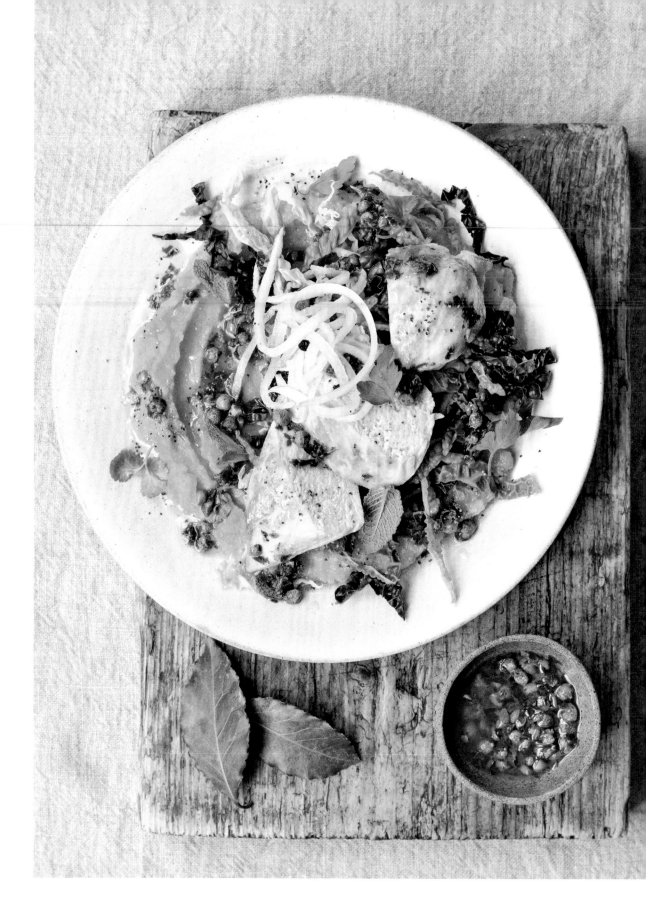

Roasted chicken breast, cavolo nero, squash purée and salsa verde

GLUTEN-FREE | DAIRY-FREE

SERVES 2

2 chicken breasts
2 tablespoons vegetable oil
150g butternut squash,
    peeled and trimmed
    weight, in even chunks
1 carrot, peeled, in even
    chunks
½ onion, finely chopped
2 garlic cloves, crushed or
    finely grated
10g coriander leaves
10g parsley leaves
5g mint leaves
20g capers
1 tablespoon olive oil
zest and juice of ½ lemon
100g (about ¼) Savoy
    cabbage, coarse ribs
    removed, leaves shredded
100g (1 bunch) cavolo nero,
    coarse stems removed,
    leaves shredded
sea salt and freshly ground
    black pepper

FOR THE
PICKLED MOOLI
1 bay leaf
½ teaspoon peppercorns
1 teaspoon caster sugar
40ml white wine vinegar
100g chunk of mooli

1   Start with the mooli. Place all the ingredients, except the mooli, in a saucepan and bring to the boil. Remove from the heat and allow to cool. Peel and julienne the mooli, then add it to the cooled pickling liquid. Leave for 1 hour to marinate.

2   Preheat the oven to 200°C (180°C fan), Gas Mark 6. Set a medium frying pan over a high heat.

3   Season the chicken and rub it with some vegetable oil, then place it in the hot frying pan and cook, turning, until golden brown on all sides. Place on a baking tray and cook in the oven for 12–15 minutes, or until cooked with no trace of pink. (If you have a probe thermometer, it's ready when it has a core temperature of 75°C.)

4   For the squash purée, place the squash and carrot chunks in a small roasting tray and toss with half the vegetable oil, salt and pepper. Roast for 10–15 minutes, turning halfway, until tender and caramelised.

5   Meanwhile, in a heavy-based saucepan, heat the remaining vegetable oil and cook the onion and garlic until softened but with no colour. Add the roast squash and carrots, pour in just enough water to cover and bring to the boil. Reduce the heat to a simmer and cook until completely tender. Strain over a bowl, retaining the liquid, then blend to a purée, adding as much liquid as you need. Season well.

6   For the sauce, blitz all the herbs with the capers and olive oil to a rough salsa. Finish with the lemon zest and juice and season to taste.

7   Bring a saucepan of water to the boil and blanch the cabbage for 2 minutes and the cavolo for 30 seconds. Drain.

8   Spoon the purée into bowls or plates and lay the drained cabbage and cavolo nero on top. Slice each chicken breast into 2–3 pieces and add to the plate with the salsa verde and pickled mooli.

Tip

Mooli (also known as daikon) is a type of radish consumed widely in Asia. Its crunchy texture makes it great for salads and stir-fries, or it's delicious pickled, as here, and used as a condiment.

NUTRITIONAL INFO PER SERVING

ENERGY 410 KCAL | FAT 22.1G | CARBS 7.7G | (OF WHICH SUGARS) 5.6G | PROTEIN 35.7G

Thai chicken curry

SERVES 2

FOR THE CURRY PASTE
2.5cm root ginger, peeled
    and roughly chopped
2 garlic cloves, roughly
    chopped
1 shallot, roughly chopped
stalks from a handful
    of coriander
1 red chilli, deseeded
2 teaspoons vegetable oil
sea salt (we use pink
    Himalayan) and freshly
    ground black pepper

FOR THE CURRY
400ml can of coconut milk
handful of lime leaves
1 lemon grass stalk, bashed
2 large chicken thighs
leaves from a handful
    of coriander
juice of ½ lemon
20g mint leaves
20g Thai basil leaves

FOR THE VEGETABLES
1 head of pak choi, finely
    sliced
100g mangetout, halved
    lengthways
100g canned bamboo
    shoots, drained, rinsed
    and sliced
1 red pepper, finely sliced

TO SERVE
lime wedges
brown rice (optional)

1   For the curry paste, put the ginger into a food processor with the garlic, shallot, coriander stalks and chilli, then blitz it all together with half the vegetable oil and some seasoning.

2   To make the curry, put the remaining 1 teaspoon oil in a heavy-based pan and fry the curry paste until you can smell that all the flavours have been released.

3   Add the coconut milk, lime leaves and lemon grass and bring the mixture to a low simmer. Add the chicken, then simmer together for a further 1–1½ hours. For the last 2 minutes of cooking time, add all the vegetables and cook until warmed through.

4   Finish with the chopped coriander leaves, then season and add the lemon juice. Scatter with the mint and Thai basil and serve with lime wedges, with brown rice on the side, if you like.

NUTRITIONAL INFO PER SERVING

ENERGY 539 KCAL | FAT 35.5G | CARBS 12.1G | (OF WHICH SUGARS) 9.1G | PROTEIN 40.2G

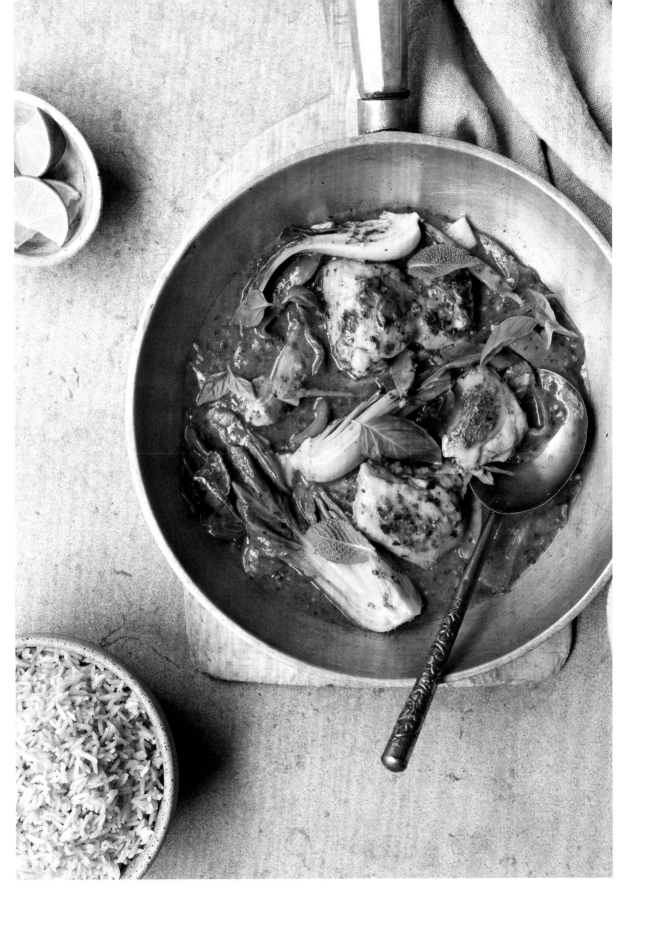

Bombay new potatoes
with spinach and tomato

VEGAN | GLUTEN-FREE | DAIRY-FREE

SERVES 2

250g new potatoes
1 tablespoon olive oil
½ teaspoon cumin seeds
½ teaspoon mustard seeds
1 shallot, finely chopped
1 garlic clove, crushed or
    finely grated
5g root ginger, peeled and
    finely grated
1 teaspoon ground
    coriander
1 teaspoon tomato purée
chilli flakes, to taste
3 tablespoons water
100g spinach
100g cherry tomatoes

1 Cut the new potatoes in half and simmer in boiling water until tender. Drain and set aside.

2 Heat the oil in a large frying pan and add the cumin seeds and mustard seeds. Cook until they start to sizzle. Add the shallot and garlic and sauté for a couple of minutes until softened. Add the ginger, coriander, tomato purée, chilli and measured water.

3 Toss in the spinach and cherry tomatoes and cook for a couple of minutes until reduced. Stir through the potatoes and cook for a final couple of minutes to bring all the ingredients together, then serve.

Tip

Using more chilli and other spices in food can be a great way to add flavour without the need for additional salt or fat.

Maple-sesame roast broccoli and cauliflower
with red chilli

VEGAN | GLUTEN-FREE | DAIRY-FREE

SERVES 2

½ head of broccoli (150g),
    cut into even florets
¼ head of cauliflower
    (150g), cut into
    even florets
1 teaspoon toasted
    sesame oil
1 tablespoon maple syrup
1 teaspoon sesame seeds,
    plus more to serve
½ red chilli, finely sliced
sea salt (we use pink
    Himalayan) and freshly
    ground black pepper

1   Preheat the oven to 220°C (200°C fan), Gas Mark 7.

2   In a large bowl, toss the broccoli and cauliflower with the sesame oil, maple syrup, sesame seeds, chilli, salt and pepper. Arrange the cauliflower florets on a non-stick baking sheet, cut sides down, if they have been halved.

3   Roast the cauliflower for 10 minutes, then add the broccoli florets and roast for a further 15 minutes, until the vegetables are tender and caramelised. Scatter with a few more sesame seeds and serve hot.

NUTRITIONAL INFO PER SERVING

ENERGY 139 KCAL | FAT 6.0G | CARBS 14.9G | (OF WHICH SUGARS) 8.0G | PROTEIN 7.5G

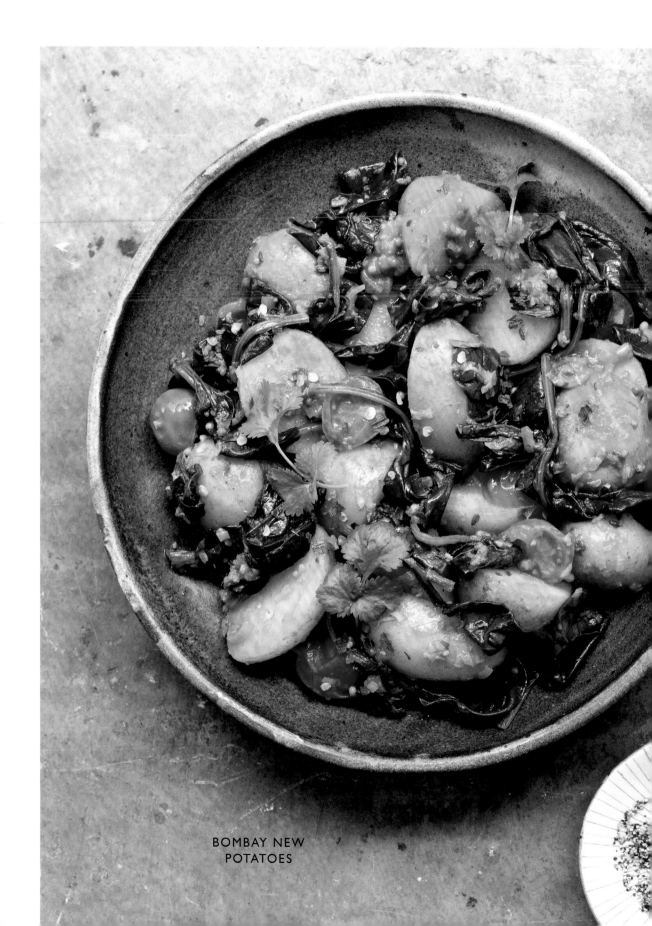

BOMBAY NEW
POTATOES

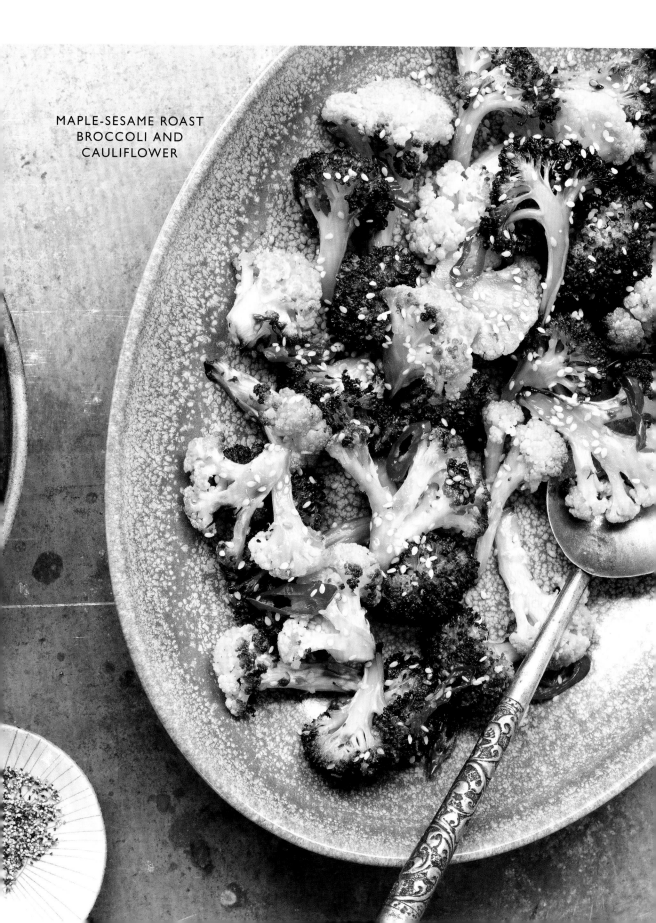

MAPLE-SESAME ROAST
BROCCOLI AND
CAULIFLOWER

Dinner
Starters

Beetroot carpaccio, whipped goat's cheese, chicory and roast pumpkin seeds

with honey-mustard dressing

VEGETARIAN (DEPENDING ON THE GOAT'S CHEESE) | GLUTEN-FREE

SERVES 4

300g raw beetroots in
   various colours
80g goat's cheese
20g cream cheese
½ garlic clove, crushed or
   finely grated
1 teaspoon finely grated
   lemon zest
30g pumpkin seeds
pinch of smoked paprika
pinch of cayenne pepper
60g chicory leaves, shredded
sea salt and freshly ground
   black pepper
micro herbs, to serve
   (optional)

FOR THE PICKLING
LIQUOR
1 tablespoon white wine
   vinegar
1 tablespoon water
½ teaspoon caster sugar
pinch of salt

FOR THE DRESSING
1 tablespoon white wine
   vinegar
2 tablespoons olive oil
2 teaspoons honey
½ teaspoon English
   mustard powder

1 Put all the ingredients for the pickling liquor in a bowl and whisk to combine. Peel half the beetroot – including all but one of the coloured varieties – slice finely on a mandolin, cover in the pickling liquor and leave for around 20 minutes. Remove from the liquor, pat dry and set aside.

2 Meanwhile, wash, peel and steam the regular (purple) beetroot and a coloured beetroot (we chose golden for the photo) for about 20 minutes until softened. Set aside to cool. Cut the cooked, cooled beetroot into a variety of slices, cubes and small wedges, to add a variation of texture and interest to the presentation.

3 In the bowl of a stand mixer (or using a bowl and an electric whisk), combine the goat's cheese, cream cheese, garlic, lemon zest and some black pepper. Blend or whip until light, then scrape into a bowl and chill.

4 Toast the pumpkin seeds in a dry pan for 2–3 minutes, then season with the pinch of smoked paprika and cayenne. Tip on to a plate and leave to cool, then roughly chop.

5 Scatter the chilled whipped goat's cheese with the seeds.

6 For the dressing, combine the white wine vinegar with the olive oil, honey and mustard powder and season. Blend well to emulsify.

7 Arrange the mixed beetroot slices, cubes and wedges attractively on 4 plates. Add chunks of the seeded whipped goat's cheese, arrange the shredded chicory on top and drizzle with the dressing. Sprinkle with micro herbs, if you like.

_____ *Tip* _____

You can use a combination
of ready-prepared natural
and pickled beetroot,
rather than buying them
raw and preparing
them yourself.

NUTRITIONAL INFO PER SERVING

ENERGY 214 KCAL | FAT 16G | CARBS 9.1G | (OF WHICH SUGARS) 7.2G | PROTEIN 7.9G

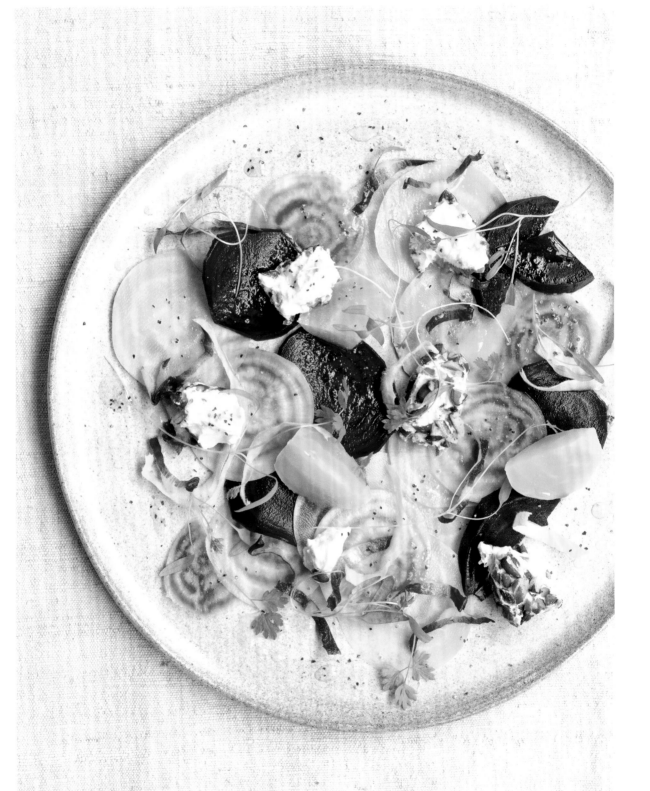

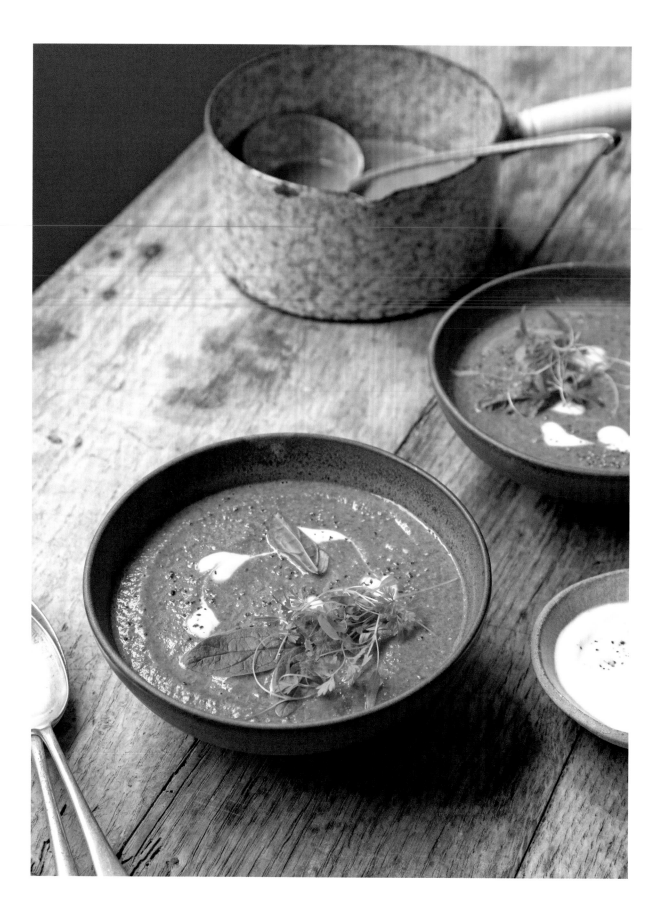

Butter bean, roast garlic and spinach soup

VEGAN | GLUTEN-FREE | DAIRY-FREE

SERVES 2

2 garlic cloves

1 teaspoon olive oil, plus
    more for the garlic

250g canned butter beans,
    drained weight, rinsed

300ml vegetable stock
    (gluten-free)

50g baby spinach

sea salt (we use pink
    Himalayan) and freshly
    ground black pepper

TO SERVE (OPTIONAL)

plant-based natural yoghurt
    (gluten-free)

handful of mixed soft herbs

1 Preheat the oven to 200°C (180°C fan), Gas Mark 6.
Brush the garlic with olive oil, seal in a foil parcel, place
on a baking tray and roast for 5–6 minutes, or until the
cloves feel soft when pressed.

2 Put the oil in a saucepan and sauté the roasted garlic
with the drained butter beans for a couple of minutes to
add colour and flavour. Pour over the vegetable stock,
bring to the boil, then reduce the heat to a simmer and
cook for 10 minutes. Add the spinach to the saucepan
to wilt down for the last couple of minutes.

3 Transfer to a blender and blitz to your desired
consistency, then taste and adjust the seasoning.
Serve, with yoghurt and soft herbs, if you like.

Tip

It's a good idea to roast
lots of garlic cloves at a
time, as the roasted pulp
is easy to freeze in small
quantities to be on hand
whenever you want it.

NUTRITIONAL INFO PER SERVING

ENERGY 117 KCAL | FAT 1.3G | CARBS 19G | (OF WHICH SUGARS) 2.0G | PROTEIN 9.5G

Vegan mozzarella and herb arancini

VEGAN | DAIRY-FREE

SERVES 2

FOR THE SAUCE

1 teaspoon olive oil

½ shallot, finely chopped

½ garlic clove, crushed or finely grated

1 teaspoon peeled and finely grated root ginger

½ red chilli, finely chopped

200g canned chopped tomatoes

sea salt (we use pink Himalayan) and freshly ground black pepper

FOR THE ARANCINI

1 teaspoon olive oil

½ shallot, finely chopped

½ garlic clove, crushed or finely chopped

80g arborio rice

200ml vegetable stock

40g vegan mozzarella, finely chopped

10g coriander leaves, finely chopped

10g parsley leaves, finely chopped

10g panko breadcrumbs

1   For the sauce, heat the oil in a heavy-based pan and sauté the shallot, garlic, ginger and chilli until soft but without colour, seasoning as you go. Add the tomatoes, bring to the boil, then reduce the heat to a simmer and cook over a low heat for 30–40 minutes. It should have a nice thick consistency. Check the seasoning, then blend until smooth.

2   To make the arancini, heat the oil in a heavy-based pan and sauté the shallot and garlic until soft but not coloured, seasoning well. Add the rice and stir until the grains are glistening with oil.

3   Add a ladle of stock and stir until it disappears. Add all the stock in this way. The process should take around 18 minutes. Spread the risotto out in a bowl and allow to cool.

4   Mix in the vegan mozzarella and the chopped herbs.

5   Meanwhile, preheat the oven to 200°C (180°C fan), Gas Mark 6.

6   With wet hands, roll the risotto into small balls (water will stop the risotto from sticking to your hands).

7   Place the panko crumbs on a tray, and roll the risotto balls in them to coat them all over. Place on a baking tray lined with baking parchment.

8   Place in the oven and cook for 15 minutes until the arancini are hot through and crisp.

9   Gently reheat the sauce, then serve the arancini with the chilli tomato sauce on the side for dipping.

NUTRITIONAL INFO PER SERVING

ENERGY 242 KCAL | FAT 8.9G | CARBS 39.2G | (OF WHICH SUGARS) 2.6G | PROTEIN 6.9G

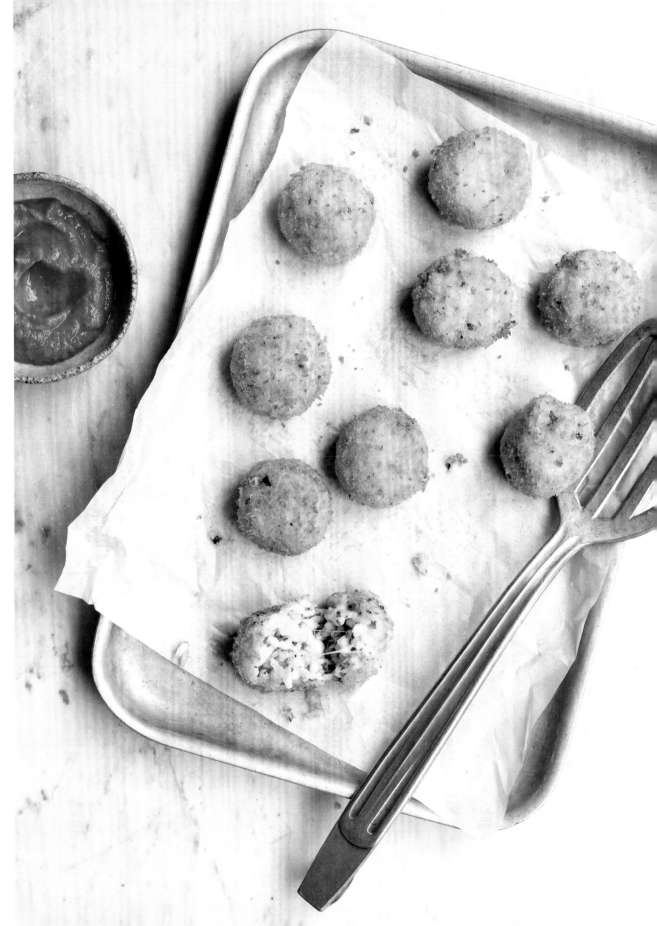

Grilled pumpkin, feta cheese, smoked almonds, parsley and mint

VEGETARIAN | GLUTEN-FREE

SERVES 2

200g pumpkin, skinned and
    trimmed weight
2 teaspoons olive oil
2 teaspoons maple syrup
20g smoked almonds
40g feta cheese (vegetarian)
10g mint leaves
10g parsley leaves
sea salt (we use pink
    Himalayan) and freshly
    ground black pepper

1   Preheat the oven to 200°C (180°C fan), Gas Mark 6.

2   Cut the pumpkin into long, thick slices, about 10cm long and 2cm thick. Lightly season them and rub with the olive oil.

3   Place an ovenproof griddle or frying pan over a high heat. Add the pumpkin slices and char them, turning to give caramelised stripes on all sides. Drizzle the slices evenly with the maple syrup, transfer to the oven and cook for 20 minutes. Remove from the oven, reserving the cooking juices.

4   Toast the smoked almonds in a hot pan for a couple of minutes, allow to cool, then roughly chop.

5   To serve, place the hot grilled pumpkin slices on 2 plates, then crumble over the feta and scatter with the smoked almonds. Sprinkle with the mint and parsley, then drizzle over the pumpkin cooking juices from the pan to finish.

Tip

Smoked almonds are a flavour bomb that bring extra protein to this dish. For a vegan version, increase the amount of almonds and leave out the feta cheese.

NUTRITIONAL INFO PER SERVING

ENERGY 307 KCAL | FAT 26.8G | CARBS 7.8G | (OF WHICH SUGARS) 3.3G | PROTEIN 9.0G

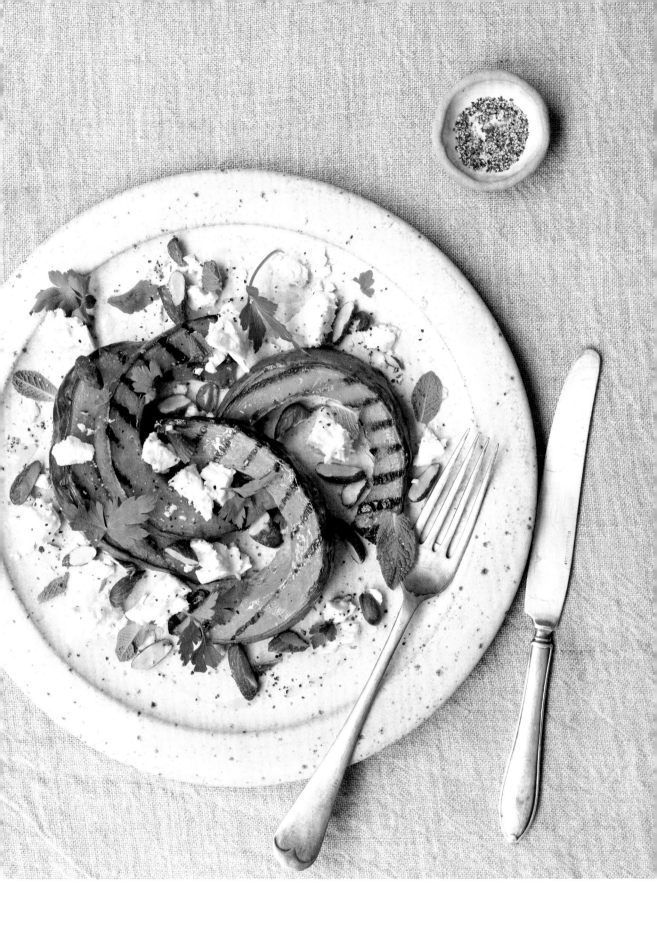

Rainbow summer rolls

*with sriracha, marinated tofu
and super seed sauce*

VEGAN | GLUTEN-FREE | DAIRY-FREE

SERVES 4

80g firm tofu, cut into strips
1 tablespoon sriracha
1½ tablespoons soy sauce
    (gluten-free), or tamari
1 teaspoon olive oil
½ large carrot
80g chunk of cucumber
    (about ¼)
60g wedge of red cabbage
½ small (40g) red pepper
½ small (40g) yellow pepper
2 spring onions
20g spinach
squeeze of lime juice
2 tablespoons chopped
    coriander leaves, plus
    more to serve
4 rice paper spring and
    summer roll wrappers
freshly ground black pepper

FOR THE SUPER SEED
SAUCE
2 tablespoons soy sauce
    (gluten-free), or tamari
2 tablespoons water
1 tablespoon sriracha
1 tablespoon pumpkin
    seed butter
½ tablespoon toasted
    sesame oil
½ tablespoon maple syrup

TO SERVE
2 teaspoons pickled ginger
    (sushi gari), to serve
sprinkle of sesame seeds,
    to serve

1   Put the tofu strips in a small bowl with the sriracha and 1 tablespoon of the soy sauce or tamari, gently stir to mix, then leave to marinate for 20–30 minutes.

2   Heat a medium frying pan and use the olive oil to fry the tofu for 4–5 minutes, turning frequently, until cooked. Set aside to cool.

3   Finely chop or shred all the vegetables and mix them together in a bowl. Add the lime juice, remaining ½ tablespoon of soy sauce or tamari and some black pepper, then mix in the coriander.

4   In a food processor, combine all the ingredients for the super seed sauce and blend well.

5   To prepare the rice paper wrappers, place each into hot water until it is soft and pliable (10–15 seconds). Blot on a clean, damp tea towel.

6   Place one-quarter of the vegetable mix and tofu in the middle of a wrapper. Fold over the bottom and sides. Roll the wrapper upwards to form a neat roll shape. Repeat to fill and form all the rolls, then refrigerate until you're ready to serve, with the dipping sauce, ginger and sesame seeds.

7   Slice the rolled wraps in half to show off their colourful filling and arrange with more coriander and a sprinkling of sesame seeds. Serve a small pot of the dipping sauce and some pickled ginger on the side.

NUTRITIONAL INFO PER SERVING

ENERGY   206 KCAL | FAT   7.6G | CARBS   25G | (OF WHICH SUGARS)   6.7G | PROTEIN   7.5G

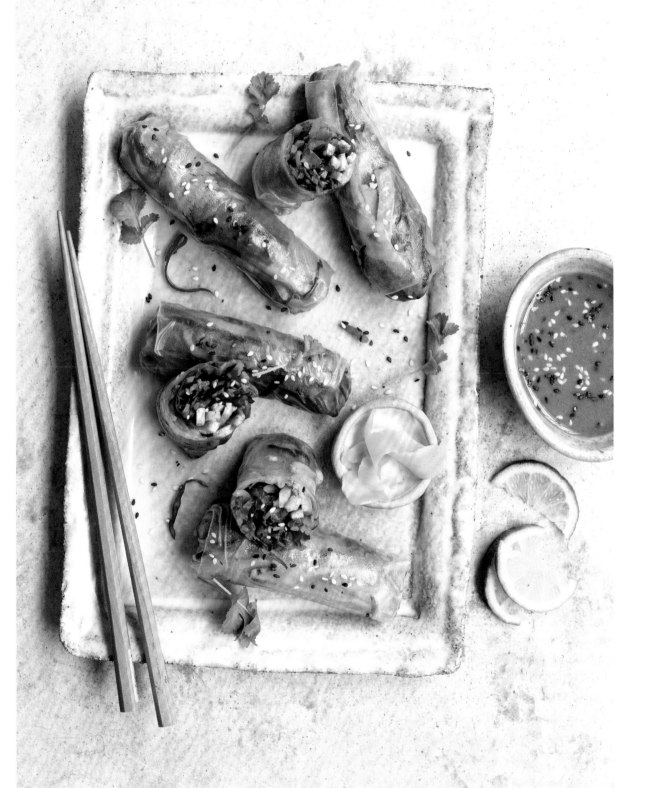

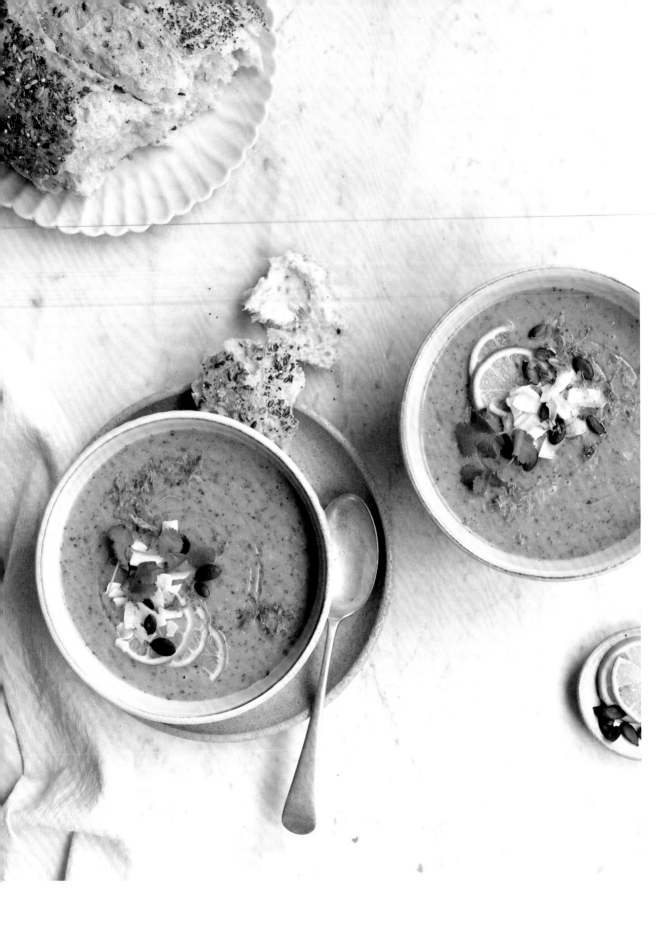

Sweet potato, coconut, lime and coriander soup

VEGAN | GLUTEN-FREE | DAIRY-FREE

SERVES 2

150g sweet potato, peeled
and chopped into
2.5cm pieces
1 teaspoon olive oil
1 medium onion, chopped
2 garlic cloves, chopped
10g root ginger, peeled
and chopped
300ml vegetable stock
(gluten-free)
100ml canned coconut milk
finely grated zest and juice
of ½ lime
large handful of coriander
leaves, plus more to serve
sea salt (we use pink
Himalayan) and freshly
ground black pepper

TO SERVE
(OPTIONAL)
coconut flakes
finely grated lime zest
lime slices
pumpkin seeds

1   Steam the sweet potato until soft. This should take about 12 minutes.

2   Heat the olive oil in a saucepan and sauté the onion, garlic and ginger, cooking for 3–4 minutes to add colour and flavour. Season well.

3   Add the sweet potato and pour over the stock and coconut milk.

4   Simmer for 10 minutes, adding the lime zest and juice and the coriander at the last minute.

5   Transfer to a blender and blitz until smooth, or to the desired consistency.

6   Serve the soup scattered with more coriander leaves, adding coconut flakes, lime zest and slices and pumpkin seeds, if you like. For a more substantial meal, serve with gluten-free bread on the side.

Tip

The natural crunch of pumpkin seeds, which are also rich in valuable omega-3 fatty acids, makes them a great finishing sprinkle for all sorts of soups and salads.

NUTRITIONAL INFO PER SERVING

ENERGY 141 KCAL | FAT 6.5G | CARBS 20.6G | (OF WHICH SUGARS) 6.9G | PROTEIN 2.5G

Smoked fish and crab cake, chipotle mayonnaise, mango-mint salad

DAIRY-FREE

SERVES 2

100g smoked haddock
100g sweet potato
1 tablespoon vegetable oil,
   plus more to oil
1 shallot, finely chopped
1 garlic clove, crushed or
   finely grated
½ teaspoon peeled and
   finely grated root ginger
100g white crab meat
5g coriander leaves
finely grated zest and juice
   of 1 lime
dash of fish sauce
100g dried breadcrumbs,
   to coat
sea salt (we use pink
   Himalayan) and freshly
   ground black pepper

FOR THE SALAD
½ mango, peeled and
   finely chopped
10g mint leaves, finely
   chopped

FOR THE MAYONNAISE
1 tablespoon light
   mayonnaise (dairy-free)
1 teaspoon chipotle paste

1   In a shallow saucepan, bring a little water to the boil, then reduce the heat to a low simmer. Add the smoked haddock and poach it until just cooked, then flake the flesh and refrigerate.

2   Bake the sweet potato in its skin until cooked (see page 66). When cool, peel and mash in a bowl.

3   Heat the oil in a saucepan and lightly sauté the shallot, garlic and ginger until they are softened but not coloured. Add to the sweet potato.

4   Mix all the ingredients for the fish cakes (except the dried breadcrumbs) together, seasoning well. Shape the mixture into 2 fish cakes, cover and chill until firm.

5   Preheat the oven to 200°C (180°C fan), Gas Mark 6.

6   For the salad, mix the mango and mint in a bowl, season well and leave to marinate for 10 minutes.

7   Mix the mayonnaise ingredients in a separate small bowl.

8   Coat the fish cakes in the crumbs, then lightly oil and season them.

9   Cook the crab cakes in the oven for 10–15 minutes until hot all the way through and golden brown. Serve with the mango-mint salad and mayo.

NUTRITIONAL INFO PER SERVING

ENERGY 184 KCAL | FAT 2.4G | CARBS 18.2G | (OF WHICH SUGARS) 4.1G | PROTEIN 23.6G

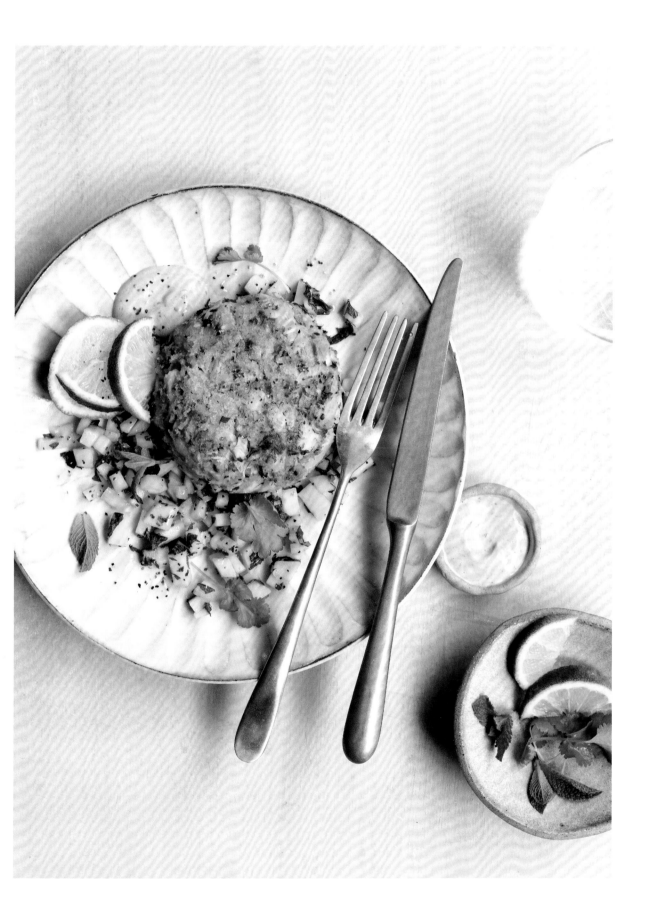

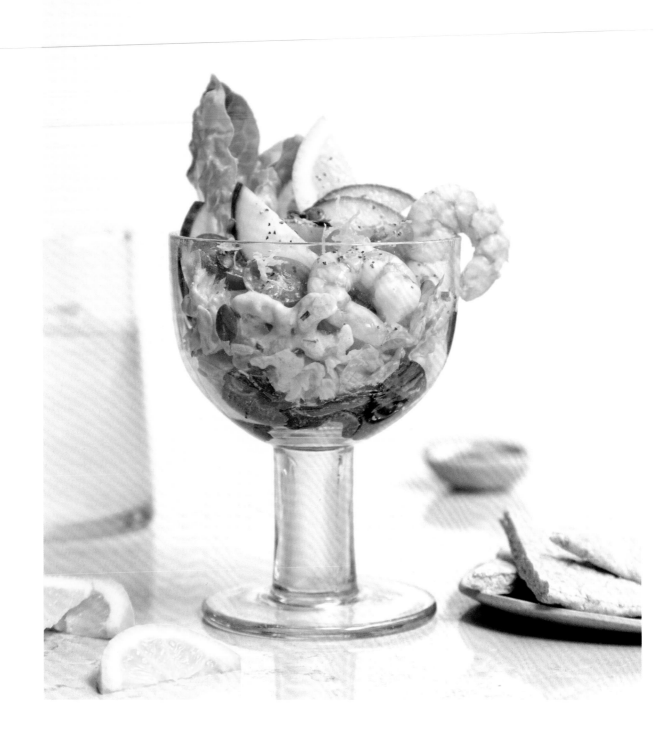

Champneys prawn cocktail

SERVES 2

a little olive oil

100g baby cherry tomatoes, halved

10cm chunk of cucumber

1 nori sheet

2 Little Gem lettuces

200g raw king prawns

2 tablespoons crème fraîche

1 tablespoon brandy

20g tomato ketchup

Tabasco sauce, to taste

1 teaspoon Worcestershire sauce

½ teaspoon paprika

5g chives, finely chopped

finely grated zest and juice of 1 lemon, plus lemon wedges to serve

100g ready-cooked small prawns

1 teaspoon toasted pumpkin seeds (see page 90)

1 wholemeal pitta bread

sea salt (we use pink Himalayan) and freshly ground black pepper

1   Lightly oil the halved cherry tomatoes and season. Separately slice the cucumber, lightly oil and season. Cut the sheet of nori into 2 squares, each just big enough to cover the bottom of a serving bowl. Separate the lettuce leaves, keeping half whole and finely slicing the rest. Set aside.

2   Bring a saucepan of lightly salted water to the boil, then reduce the heat to a low simmer. Gently poach the king prawns for 4–5 minutes, then drain them, put on a plate, cover and refrigerate.

3   To make the sauce, in a small mixing bowl combine the crème fraîche, brandy, ketchup, Tabasco and Worcestershire sauces, paprika, chives and lemon juice and season.

4   Put the nori into 2 serving bowls and add the sliced lettuce. Arrange over the small prawns with a couple of spoons of the sauce. Arrange the king prawns on top and scatter with the tomatoes and cucumber, pumpkin seeds and lemon zest. Place the whole lettuce leaves to the side of each prawn cocktail.

5   Toast the pitta bread, then cut into triangles. Serve the pitta triangles and lemon wedges with the prawn cocktails.

NUTRITIONAL INFO PER SERVING

ENERGY 327 KCAL | FAT 9.6G | CARBS 26.9G | (OF WHICH SUGARS) 10.9G | PROTEIN 31.6G

Seared scallops, curried parsnip purée, pickled raisins, parsnip crisps

GLUTEN-FREE | DAIRY-FREE

SERVES 2

1 small parsnip (100g)

2 teaspoons olive oil, plus more for the crisps

10g cashew nuts

1 teaspoon curry powder (gluten-free)

1 garlic clove, finely chopped

1 shallot, finely chopped

½ teaspoon peeled and finely grated root ginger

1 teaspoon ground coriander

leaves from 2 large coriander sprigs, chopped

½ lemon

250g large scallops

1 teaspoon coconut flakes, toasted

sea salt (we use pink Himalayan) and freshly ground black pepper

FOR THE PICKLED RAISINS

200ml water

2 teaspoons maple syrup

1 teaspoon apple cider vinegar

10g raisins

1 For the pickled raisins, pour the measured water into a saucepan and add the maple syrup and vinegar. Bring to the boil, remove from the heat and add the raisins. Set aside to soak for 2–3 hours.

2 Preheat the oven to 120°C (100°C fan), Gas Mark ½.

3 For the parsnip crisps and purée, scrub the parsnip very well. Peel it – reserving the peelings – then cut the parsnip into even-sized pieces. Boil the pieces in salted water until very soft, then strain over a bowl, keeping the cooking liquor.

4 Meanwhile, lightly oil the parsnip peelings, place on a baking tray and cook in the low oven until crisp.

5 Tip the cashew nuts into a dry pan and dry-fry until toasted, adding half the curry powder, salt and pepper to add flavour, then tip out on to a plate.

6 Heat 1 teaspoon of the oil in a heavy-based pan and sauté the garlic, shallot and ginger until soft, seasoning lightly. Add the remaining curry powder and the ground coriander and cook for a further few minutes. Sprinkle with some of the chopped coriander, then set aside and allow to cool.

7 Place the shallot mix and boiled parsnip in a blender and blitz, gradually adding some of the cooking liquor until you reach the desired consistency. Season, adding a squeeze of lemon juice for acidity.

8 Now for the scallops. Dab them dry with kitchen paper, then season each well. Add the remaining oil to a smoking-hot pan over a very high heat. Add the scallops and cook until golden brown on the bases, then turn and immediately remove the pan from the heat. Leave the scallops to cook in the residual heat for 2–3 minutes, depending on size.

9 Decorate the plates with the curried parsnip purée, then add the scallops. Scatter with the pickled raisins, curried toasted cashews and toasted coconut, then serve sprinkled with the parsnip crisps and remaining coriander leaves.

NUTRITIONAL INFO PER SERVING

ENERGY 223 KCAL | FAT 10.3G | CARBS 15.8G | (OF WHICH SUGARS) 5.5G | PROTEIN 16.1G

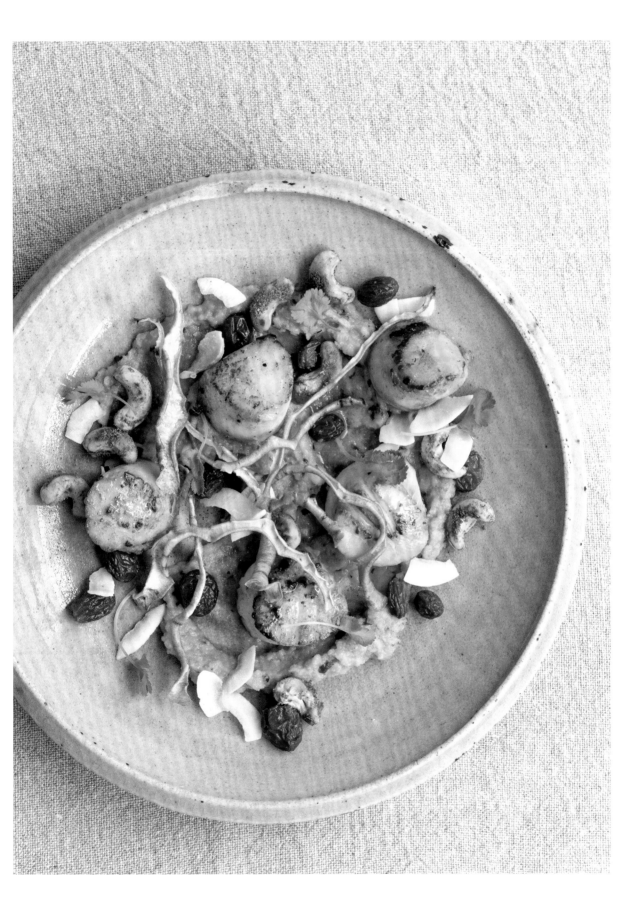

Sticky beef teriyaki
with shredded vegetables

DAIRY-FREE

SERVES 2

FOR THE BEEF AND STICKY SAUCE

1 teaspoon runny honey

25ml soy sauce

50ml teriyaki sauce

1 teaspoon ground
   coriander

5g root ginger, peeled
   and finely grated

1 garlic clove, crushed
   or finely grated

200g bavette steak,
   thinly sliced

sea salt (we use pink
   Himalayan)

sesame seeds, to serve

FOR THE VEGETABLES

1 teaspoon olive oil

5g root ginger, peeled and
   finely grated

1 garlic clove, finely sliced

1 spring onion, finely sliced

1 bunch (100g) kale, weight
   with coarse stems
   removed, leaves shredded

1 bunch (100g) cavolo nero,
   weight with coarse stems
   removed, leaves shredded

mixed shredded vegetables
   (carrots, mixed pepper,
   spring onions), to serve

1   Combine all the ingredients for the sauce, except the steak and sesame seeds, in a bowl, season with salt, stir in the meat, cover and let it soak up the flavours for 4–6 hours.

2   Heat the olive oil in a wok or deep frying pan and sauté the ginger and garlic with a pinch of salt until fragrant, then add the spring onion and cook until it starts to soften.

3   Remove the beef strips from the marinade, reserving the sauce, and stir-fry the meat for 3–4 minutes. Add the sauce and cook over a high heat for a further 2 minutes, so the sauce reduces and becomes sticky. Remove the beef from the pan, then set aside to rest.

4   Add the kale and cavolo nero to the pan and cook for a couple of minutes until tender. Divide between 2 bowls.

5   Place the beef on the greens. Add the shredded vegetables and drizzle over any remaining sauce, then sprinkle with sesame seeds to serve.

Tip

To make this a more substantial meal, serve with wholegrain rice.

NUTRITIONAL INFO PER SERVING

ENERGY 336 KCAL | FAT 18.2G | CARBS 17.6G | (OF WHICH SUGARS) 16G | PROTEIN 26.6G

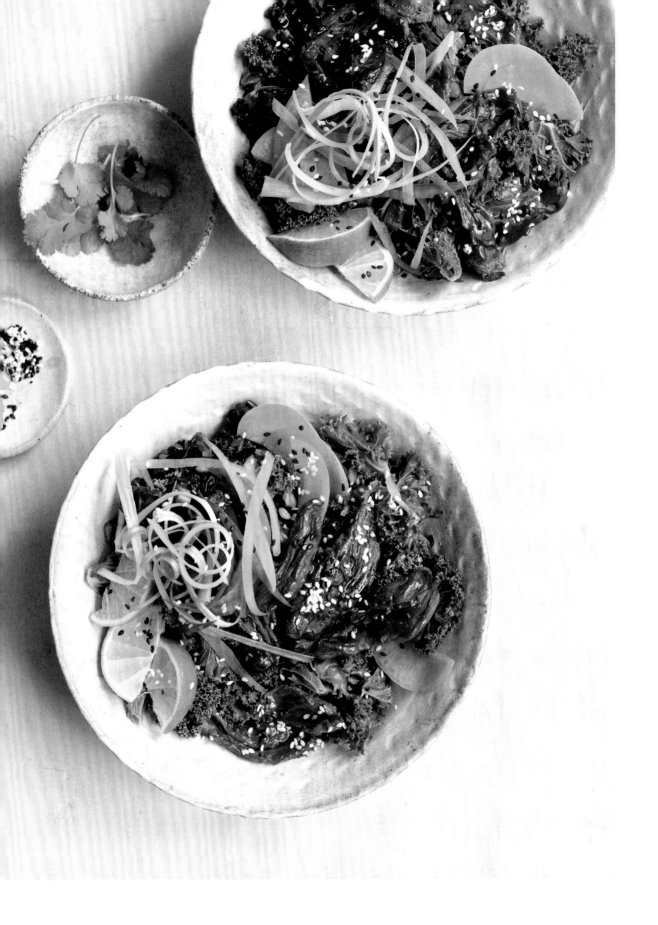

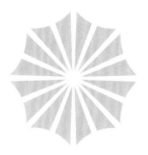

Dinner
Main
Courses

Green lentil and sweet potato cottage pie

VEGAN | GLUTEN-FREE | DAIRY-FREE

SERVES 2

1 teaspoon olive oil

1 medium onion, finely
chopped

1 medium carrot (100g),
finely chopped

2 celery sticks (100g),
finely chopped

1 garlic clove, crushed or
finely grated

150ml vegetable stock
(gluten-free)

1 teaspoon red wine vinegar

50ml tomato juice

1 teaspoon chopped
thyme leaves

1 teaspoon tomato purée
(gluten-free)

1 teaspoon tamari

½ teaspoon maple syrup

200g canned green lentils,
drained weight, rinsed

200g canned chopped
tomatoes

100ml water

sprinkle of pumpkin seeds

sea salt (we use pink
Himalayan) and freshly
ground black pepper

steamed broccoli and kale,
to serve

FOR THE MASH

200g sweet potato,
finely chopped

10g plant-based spread
(gluten-free)

1 teaspoon Dijon mustard

2 tablespoons unsweetened
soya milk

1 Heat a large saucepan with the olive oil over
a medium heat. Add the onion, carrot and celery and
cook for 8–10 minutes until softened but not coloured,
then add the garlic and cook for another minute.

2 In a jug, mix the vegetable stock with the red wine
vinegar and tomato juice. Pour in the mixture to
deglaze the pan, scraping up bits stuck on the bottom,
and simmer for 2 minutes until most of the liquid has
evaporated. Stir in the thyme, tomato purée, tamari
and maple syrup.

3 Tip in the lentils, chopped tomatoes and measured
water and simmer for 10–12 minutes until the sauce has
reduced and is thick enough to coat the back of a spoon.

4 Meanwhile, make the mash topping. Bring a large
pan of water to the boil, add the sweet potato and
simmer for 10–15 minutes until cooked all the way
through. Drain, then add the dairy-free spread,
mustard and soya milk and mash until smooth,
then season to taste.

5 Preheat the oven to 200°C (180°C fan), Gas Mark 6.

6 Season the filling, pour it into a small oven dish and
allow to cool slightly. Top with the mash, starting with
spoonfuls on the outside corners and working your way
inwards, so the filling doesn't spill out. Sprinkle the
pumpkin seeds on top and bake for 30–35 minutes until
golden and bubbling.

7 Serve with steamed broccoli and kale.

NUTRITIONAL INFO PER SERVING

ENERGY 327 KCAL | FAT 6.8G | CARBS 51.8G | (OF WHICH SUGARS) 15.6G | PROTEIN 17.5G

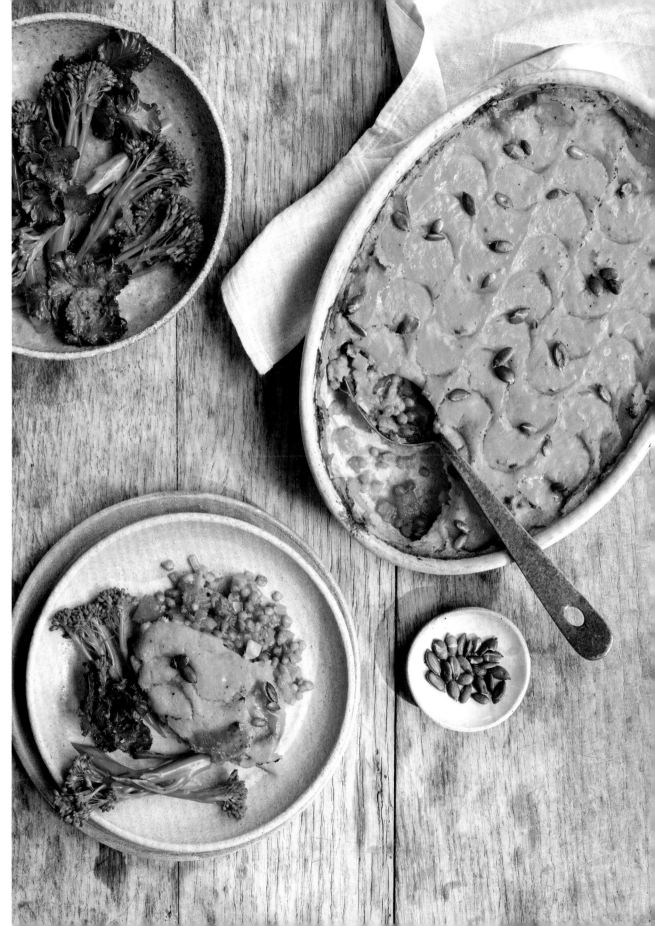

Mexicana black bean lettuce cups

VEGAN | GLUTEN-FREE | DAIRY-FREE

SERVES 2

olive oil spray

150g plant-based mince
   (gluten-free)

150g canned black beans,
   drained weight, rinsed

10g fajita seasoning
   (gluten-free)

1 garlic clove, crushed or
   finely grated

1 red pepper, or ½ each
   red and yellow pepper
   (100g total weight),
   finely chopped

100g mushrooms,
   finely chopped

1 medium carrot (100g),
   finely chopped

½ courgette (100g),
   finely chopped

1 onion, finely chopped

1 Iceberg lettuce, leaves
   separated

10g coriander leaves

FOR THE DIP

50g natural soya yoghurt
   (gluten-free)

10g chives, finely chopped

finely grated zest of
   1 lime

**FOR THE TOMATO
SALSA**

1 large plum tomato,
   finely chopped

¼ red onion, finely chopped

1 teaspoon finely chopped
   pickled jalapeños

leaves from 1 coriander
   sprig, chopped

finely grated zest and juice
   of ½ lime

pinch each of ground cumin,
   dried oregano, sea salt
   (we use pink Himalayan)
   and freshly ground
   black pepper

1   Spray a sauté pan with olive oil spray and sauté the plant-based mince, black beans and half the fajita seasoning until warmed through and well combined, or according to the packet instructions for the mince. Turn off the heat and set aside.

2   Sauté the garlic and all the vegetables, except the lettuce, in a little more olive oil spray and the remaining fajita seasoning, cooking until they are softened but without colour. Add the cooked mince and beans.

3   In a small bowl, combine all the ingredients for the soya yoghurt dip. In a separate bowl, combine all the ingredients for the tomato salsa.

4   Serve the mince and vegetables in Iceberg lettuce leaf bowls with the coriander, with small bowls of the tomato salsa and yoghurt dip.

NUTRITIONAL INFO PER SERVING

ENERGY 280 KCAL | FAT 7.4G | CARBS 34.7G | (OF WHICH SUGARS) 18G | PROTEIN 22.8G

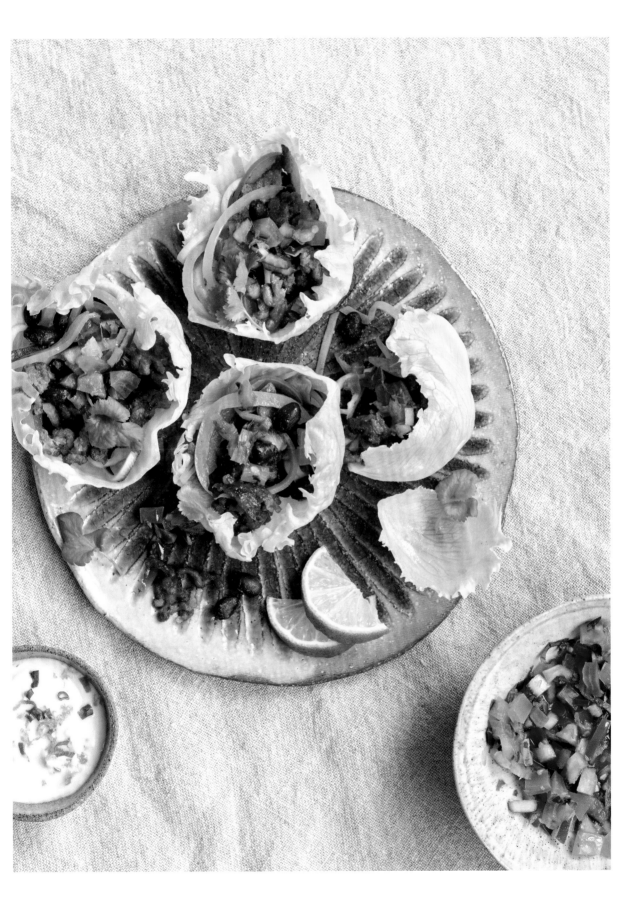

Rainbow soul bowl

VEGAN | GLUTEN-FREE | DAIRY-FREE

SERVES 2

120g smoked tofu
2 tablespoons olive oil
finely grated zest and juice
    of 1 lime
½ teaspoon chipotle chilli
    paste (gluten-free)
2 tablespoons soy sauce
    (gluten-free), or tamari
2 teaspoons maple syrup
olive oil spray
80g butternut squash,
    peeled, deseeded
120g Tenderstem broccoli
10g pumpkin seeds
garlic powder (gluten-free)
1 avocado
juice of 1 lemon or lime
80g roasted red pepper
    from a jar, sliced

80g canned sweetcorn,
    drained weight, rinsed
80g canned black beans,
    drained weight, rinsed
100g sauerkraut
    (unpasteurised)
40g pomegranate seeds
sea salt (we use pink
    Himalayan) and freshly
    ground black pepper

1   Cut the tofu into bite-sized cubes (1–2cm). In a mixing bowl, combine the olive oil, lime zest and juice, chipotle paste, soy sauce and maple syrup. Add the tofu and gently stir to coat. Cover and leave to marinate for at least 5–10 minutes, but ideally 1–2 hours.

2   Heat a wok or large frying pan over a medium heat.

3   Remove the tofu from the marinade, setting the marinade aside. Fry the tofu in olive oil spray for 5–10 minutes until golden brown all over, then set aside. Strain the marinade to remove any small pieces of tofu.

4   Cut the butternut squash into cubes the same size as the tofu. Steam for 5–6 minutes. Mist the wok or frying pan with more olive oil spray and cook the squash cubes with a drizzle of the tofu marinade for a further 2–3 minutes until softened but still with a little bite. Set aside.

NUTRITIONAL INFO PER SERVING

ENERGY   467 KCAL | FAT   28G | CARBS   30G | (OF WHICH SUGARS) 20G | PROTEIN   18G

5 Trim the broccoli and steam until al dente. Transfer to iced water to stop the cooking. Drain very well.

6 Toast the pumpkin seeds in the frying pan with a little seasoning and garlic powder, then tip on to a plate and set aside.

7 Peel and remove the stone from the avocado, then thickly slice it. Dress with lemon or lime juice to stop it browning and season with salt and pepper.

8 Arrange all the elements in colour wheel-order: first red pepper, then squash, sweetcorn, avocado, broccoli and black beans, finishing with the tofu cubes.

9 Shake the remaining tofu marinade to revive and emulsify it, then use it to dress the dish.

10 Serve with the sauerkraut, sprinkling over the pumpkin and pomegranate seeds to finish.

_____ *Tip* _____

Choose unpasteurised sauerkraut for higher levels of live micro-organisms.

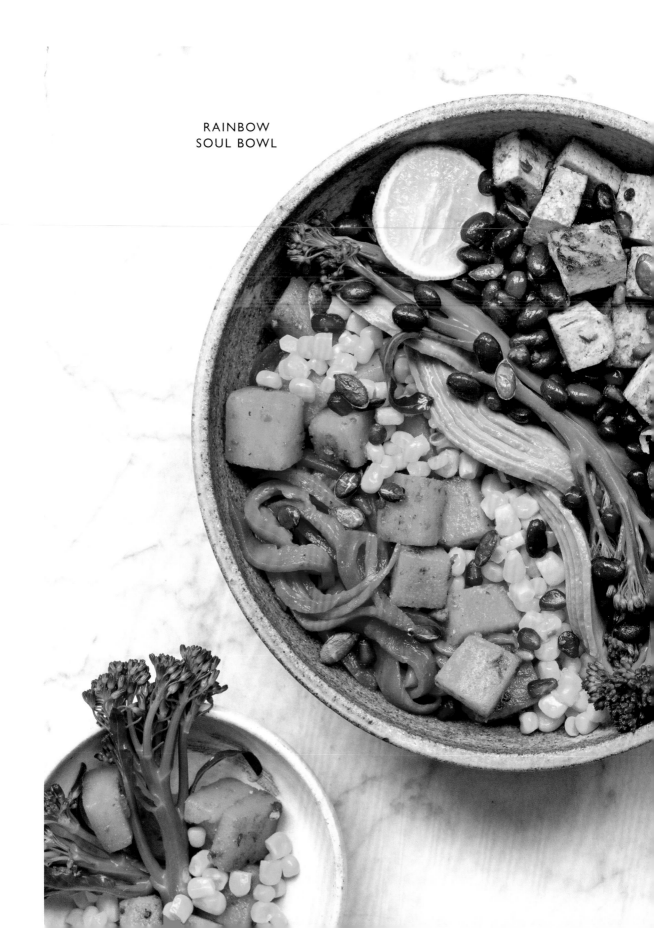

RAINBOW
SOUL BOWL

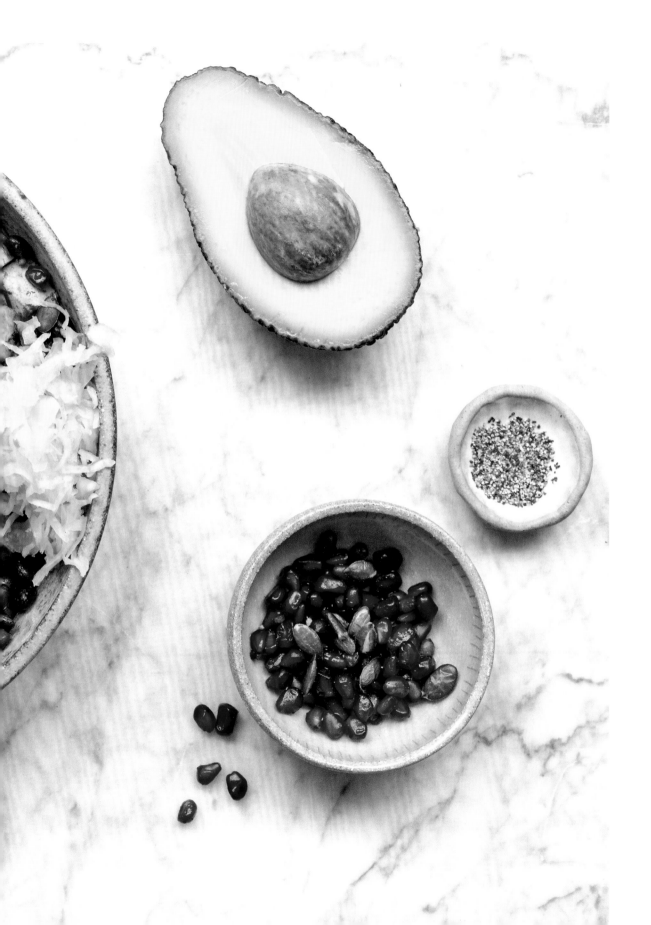

Thai red butter bean curry
with pumpkin seeds and coriander

VEGAN | GLUTEN-FREE | DAIRY-FREE

SERVES 2

½ medium butternut
squash, peeled,
deseeded and chopped
into 2.5cm cubes
1 medium onion,
finely chopped
1 garlic clove, crushed or
finely grated
1 teaspoon coconut oil
(we use raw organic
extra-virgin)
200g canned butter beans,
drained weight, rinsed
150g frozen peas, defrosted
150ml unsweetened
coconut drinking milk
2 tablespoons Thai red
curry paste (gluten-free)
1 red pepper, finely chopped
100g spinach
1 red chilli, finely chopped
200g green beans, chopped
finely grated zest of 1 lime
10g pumpkin seeds
large handful of coriander
leaves

TO SERVE (OPTIONAL)
1 tablespoon desiccated
coconut
brown rice

1 Put the squash cubes in a steamer and steam until al dente, which should take 6–7 minutes, but check they are tender to the point of a knife. Set aside.

2 Fry the onion and garlic in the coconut oil for 5 minutes, continually stirring. Start over a high heat, then reduce it to medium, so the onions brown well, but without burning. Add the squash, butter beans and peas and cook for another minute.

3 Next, blend the coconut milk with the curry paste and and add to the squash mixture, making sure everything is well coated. Simmer for 10 minutes, uncovered, so the sauce thickens and reduces.

4 Pop in the red pepper and spinach and cook for 2 minutes more. Check the seasoning, adding a little of the chilli if necessary to achieve a medium–spicy, rich flavour.

5 Meanwhile, steam the green beans for a couple of minutes until al dente.

6 Serve the curry over a bed of the chopped green beans, sprinkled with the remaining red chilli, lime zest, pumpkin seeds and coriander leaves, adding the desiccated coconut, if you like. Offer brown rice on the side, for those who want it.

NUTRITIONAL INFO PER SERVING

ENERGY 409 KCAL | FAT 14.2G | CARBS 56.9G | (OF WHICH SUGARS) 18.3G | PROTEIN 23.8G

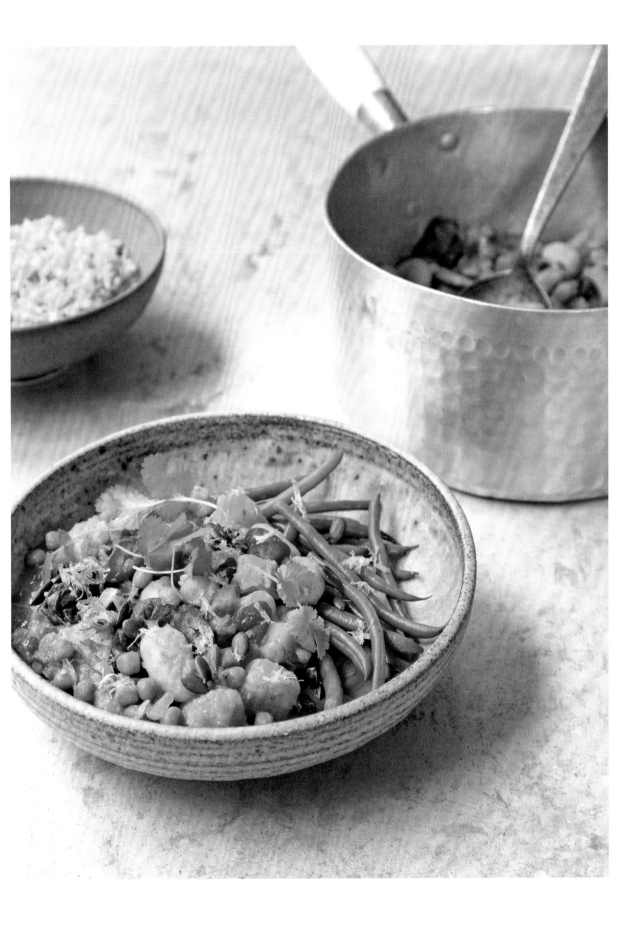

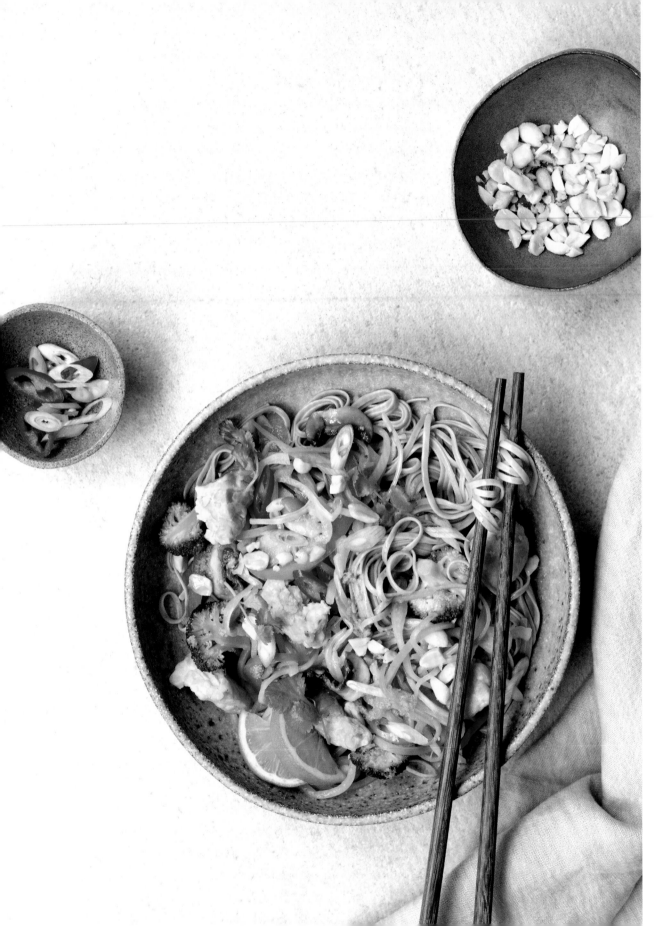

Tempeh chow mein
with buckwheat noodles and peanuts

VEGAN | GLUTEN-FREE | DAIRY-FREE

SERVES 2

100g buckwheat soba
   noodles (gluten-free)

2 tablespoons soy sauce
   (gluten-free), or tamari

10g root ginger, peeled and
   finely grated

2 garlic cloves, crushed or
   finely grated

2 teaspoons maple syrup

2 teaspoons rice wine
   vinegar

olive oil spray

200g tempeh

about ¼ small white
   cabbage (100g), shredded

2 medium-small carrots
   (100g), shredded

100g mushrooms, sliced

80g beansprouts

1 red pepper, finely sliced

about ½ small head of
   broccoli (150g), cut into
   small florets

10g peanuts, roughly
   chopped

2 spring onions, finely sliced

TO SERVE
coriander leaves
red chilli, finely sliced
lime slices

1 Prepare the noodles according to the packet instructions.

2 In a small bowl, whisk together the soy sauce or tamari, ginger, garlic, maple syrup and rice wine vinegar.

3 Place a large wok over a medium-high heat and mist it with olive oil spray. Add the tempeh, crumbling it between your fingers, then cook for 2 minutes.

4 Add the cabbage, carrots, mushrooms, beansprouts, pepper and broccoli and pour three-quarters of the sauce over the top. Stir-fry, mixing well, for another 5–7 minutes, stirring occasionally, until the cabbage has shrunk down and softened.

5 Add the noodles, peanuts, spring onions and remaining sauce, toss to coat, then continue cooking until the noodles are warmed through. Season to taste and serve with coriander leaves, red chilli and lime slices.

NUTRITIONAL INFO PER SERVING

ENERGY 430 KCAL | FAT 9.2G | CARBS 67.5G | (OF WHICH SUGARS) 15.8G | PROTEIN 22.9G

Baked salmon, butter bean cassoulet, saffron velouté

GLUTEN-FREE

SERVES 4

about 2 banana shallots
(50g), finely chopped

1 large garlic clove,
finely chopped

20ml rapeseed oil

about ½ leek (50g), sliced
into half moons

1 medium-small carrot
(50g), finely chopped

200ml vegetable stock
(gluten-free)

1 bay leaf

2 thyme sprigs

4 x 140g salmon fillets

200g canned butter beans,
drained weight, rinsed

5g parsley leaves,
roughly chopped

5g tarragon leaves,
finely chopped

sea salt (we use pink
Himalayan) and freshly
ground black pepper

FOR THE SAFFRON
VELOUTÉ

1 large banana shallot,
finely chopped

50ml dry white wine

100ml fish stock
(gluten-free)

150ml double cream

pinch of saffron strands
or powder

juice of ½ lemon

1   Start with the cassoulet. Lightly sauté the shallots and garlic in half the oil over a medium heat, until softened but not coloured. Add the leek and carrot and cook for a further 5 minutes. Pour in the stock, add the bay and thyme and cook for 2–3 minutes until the vegetables are tender, but not overcooked.

2   Preheat the oven to 200°C (180°C fan), Gas Mark 6.

3   Season the salmon fillets and lightly rub them with a little of the remaining oil, place on a baking tray lined with baking parchment and cook for 8 minutes. Remove from the oven and rest for 2 minutes.

4   Meanwhile, make the velouté. Slowly cook the shallot in the remaining oil until softened but not coloured. Pour in the wine and reduce the liquid until almost completely evaporated. Pour in the fish stock and reduce by half. Add the cream and saffron, then reduce to a velvety texture and season well. Pass through a sieve, then season with the lemon juice.

5   Add the butter beans to the cassoulet along with the herbs. Bring to the boil, then season to taste.

6   Serve the salmon and cassoulet with the saffron velouté on the side.

NUTRITIONAL INFO PER SERVING

ENERGY 453 KCAL | FAT 26.9G | CARBS 11.1G | (OF WHICH SUGARS) 5.2G | PROTEIN 41.2G

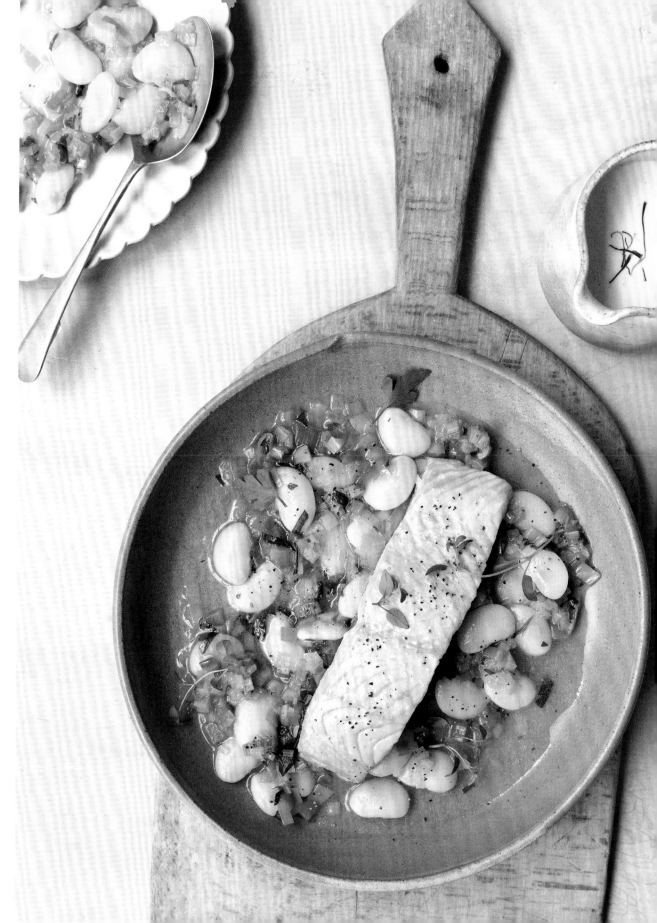

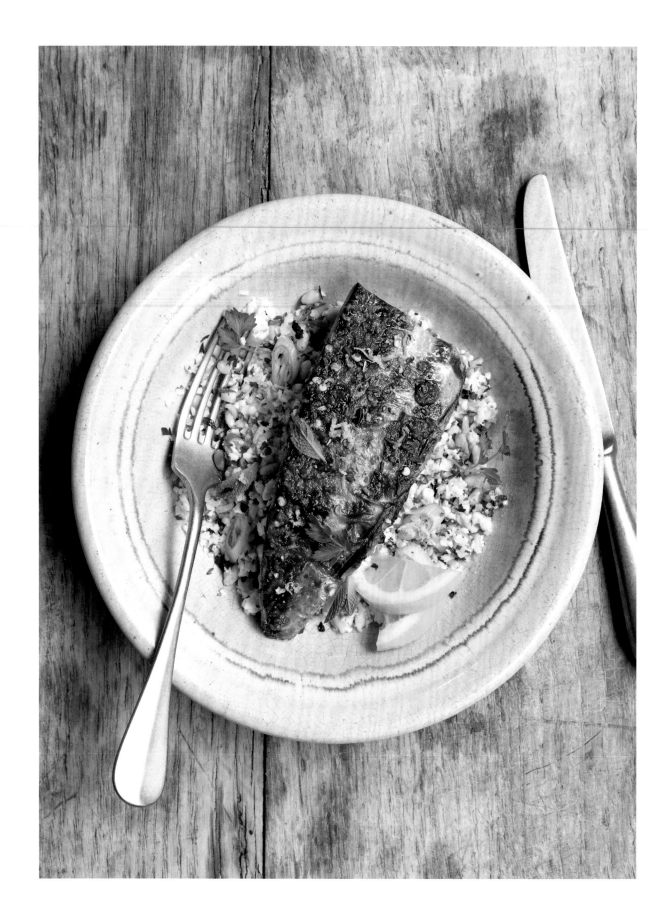

Peri peri mackerel, lemon and parsley cauliflower wild rice

GLUTEN-FREE | DAIRY-FREE

SERVES 2

50g wild rice
1 tablespoon tomato purée
1 teaspoon peri peri
    seasoning (gluten-free),
    plus more to serve
2 large mackerel fillets
½ medium cauliflower,
    broken into florets
2 tablespoons olive oil
2 spring onions, finely sliced
2 teaspoons pine nuts
1 bunch of parsley, leaves
    chopped
large handful of mint leaves,
    chopped
finely grated zest and juice
    of 1 lemon, plus more
    zest to serve
50ml canned coconut milk
sea salt (we use pink
    Himalayan) and freshly
    ground black pepper

1   Cook the wild rice according to the packet instructions, then set aside.

2   Combine the tomato purée with the peri peri seasoning and rub the mixture over the mackerel.

3   Place the cauliflower in a food processor with 1 tablespoon of the olive oil, salt and pepper and pulse until broken down into rice-sized pieces. Do not let the food processor run, or you'll end up with white mush. Mix the cauliflower rice with the cooled wild rice, sliced spring onions, pine nuts, most of the parsley and mint, the lemon zest and juice, coconut milk and salt and pepper to taste.

4   Heat the remaining 1 tablespoon olive oil in a frying pan over a high heat and sauté the fish, skin side down, for 3–4 minutes, then flip and cook for a further few minutes, ensuring it is cooked through (the flesh should lose its translucency and turn opaque throughout the fillets).

5   Serve the mackerel on a bed of the cauliflower wild rice and sprinkle with the remaining parsley and mint, then scatter with lemon zest and add a little pinch of the peri peri seasoning to taste.

NUTRITIONAL INFO PER SERVING

ENERGY 521 KCAL | FAT 35G | CARBS 30G | (OF WHICH SUGARS) 8.8G | PROTEIN 25.4G

Prawn and vegetable ramen
with ginger soy broth and glass noodles

GLUTEN-FREE | DAIRY-FREE

SERVES 4

200ml vegetable stock
(gluten-free)
5g root ginger, peeled and
finely grated
3g coriander stalks, finely
chopped
1 lime leaf, finely chopped
lime juice, to taste
soy sauce (gluten-free), or
tamari, to taste
½ teaspoon cornflour
1 bunch of spring onions,
finely chopped, plus more
to serve
200g rice noodles
1 tablespoon coconut oil
(we use raw organic
extra-virgin)
500g tiger prawns
½ large bunch (60g) cavolo
nero, weight with coarse
ribs removed, shredded
1 small head of pak choi, cut
into very slim wedges
handful of beansprouts
1 red chilli, finely chopped
the leaves from the
coriander stalks in
the broth
lime wedges, to serve

1 Pour the stock into a saucepan and add the ginger, coriander stalks and lime leaf. Taste and season with the lime juice and soy sauce or tamari.

2 Mix the cornflour in a cup with a little water until smooth, then stir into the broth. The broth should thicken to the consistency of single cream. Pass it through a sieve into a clean saucepan, then add the spring onions.

3 Soak the rice noodles according to the packet instructions (usually 2–3 minutes).

4 Heat the oil in a large saucepan or wok and stir-fry the prawns, cavolo nero and pak choi for a minute. Pour in the broth and bring to the boil, then add the drained noodles and beansprouts to the pan or wok.

5 Divide between bowls, scatter with red chilli slices, shredded spring onions and coriander leaves and serve with lime wedges.

Tip

Save vegetable trimmings in a bag in the freezer, then make a big pot of vegetable stock when you have collected enough. It's a great base for all broths and soups, and more nutritious than instant versions.

NUTRITIONAL INFO PER SERVING

ENERGY 332 KCAL | FAT 6.9G | CARBS 42.5G | (OF WHICH SUGARS) 8.3G | PROTEIN 22.1G

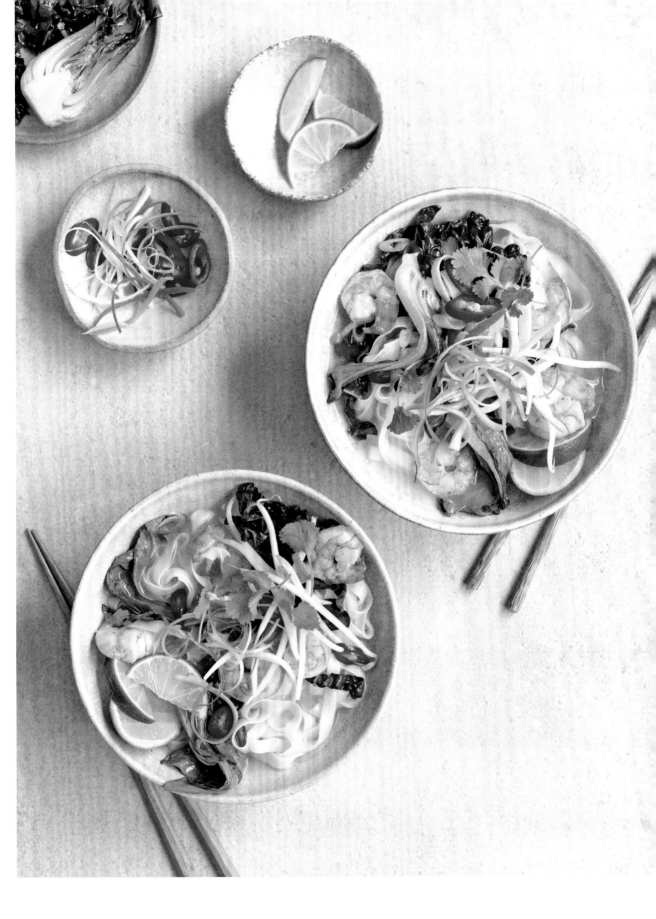

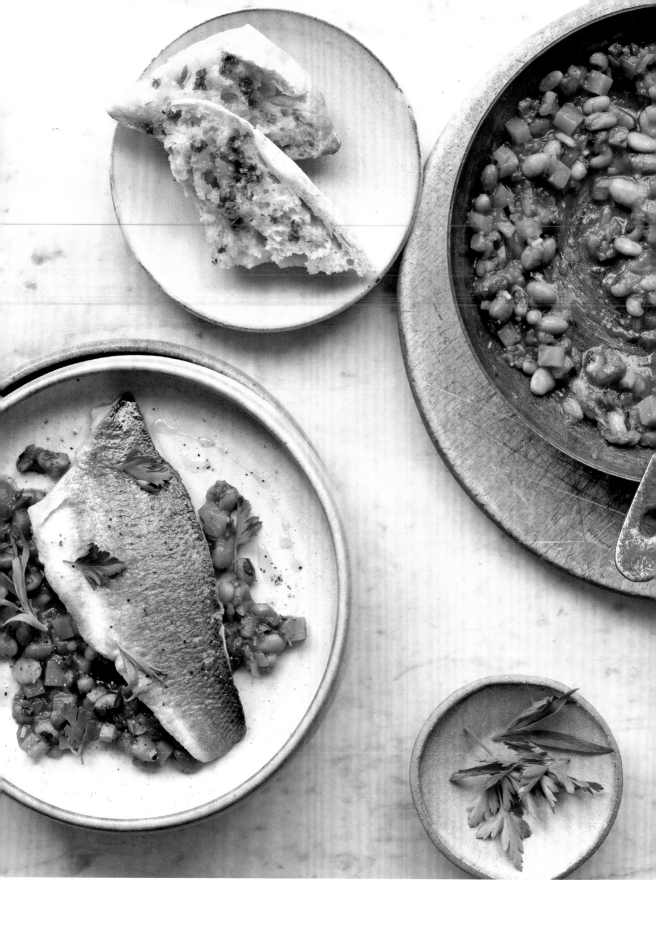

Sea bass
with mixed beans

GLUTEN-FREE | DAIRY-FREE

SERVES 4

1 tablespoon extra-virgin
    rapeseed oil, plus more
    for the fish
½ small red onion (50g),
    finely chopped
1 large garlic clove, crushed
    or finely grated
1 medium-small carrot
    (50g), finely chopped
100g chopped tomatoes
100ml vegetable stock
    (gluten-free)
½ teaspoon thyme leaves
75g canned mixed beans,
    drained weight, rinsed
4 x 140g sea bass fillets
5g tarragon leaves, chopped
5g parsley leaves, chopped
sea salt (we use pink
    Himalayan) and freshly
    ground black pepper

1   Heat the oil in a saucepan and sauté the red onion and garlic until softened, but not coloured. Add the carrot and cook for a further 5 minutes. Pour in the tomatoes and stock and bring to the boil. Reduce the heat to a simmer, add the thyme and beans, cover and simmer over a gentle heat for 40 minutes.

2   Preheat the oven to 200°C (180°C fan), Gas Mark 6.

3   Season the fish fillets and oil them well. Set on a baking sheet lined with baking parchment and place in the oven for 6 minutes. Remove and leave to rest for 2 minutes.

4   Season the beans, add the tarragon and parsley, then serve the beans with the sea bass.

Tip

You could also try this recipe with other fish fillets instead of sea bass. Basa is widely sold and useful to have stashed in the freezer.

NUTRITIONAL INFO PER SERVING

ENERGY 322 KCAL | FAT 8.5G | CARBS 18.6G | (OF WHICH SUGARS) 7.7G | PROTEIN 25.5G

Baked hake, dill potato crush, tartare cream and samphire

GLUTEN-FREE

SERVES 4

FOR THE POTATO CRUSH
400g new potatoes
5g dill, chopped
6 spring onions,
  finely shredded
2 teaspoons extra-virgin
  rapeseed oil
sea salt (we use pink
  Himalayan) and freshly
  ground black pepper

FOR THE CREAM
1 tablespoon vegetable oil
about 2 banana shallots (50g),
  finely chopped
1 large garlic clove,
  finely chopped
50ml dry white wine
100ml fish stock (gluten-free)
100ml double cream
15g capers
15g cornichons, finely
  chopped
5g parsley leaves, chopped
juice of 1 lemon

**FOR THE FISH
AND SAMPHIRE**
4 x 140g hake fillets
extra-virgin rapeseed oil
50g samphire

1 Boil the new potatoes in salted water until soft, then drain and place in a mixing bowl. Lightly crush the potatoes with a large fork, adding the dill, spring onions and rapeseed oil. Mix gently and season. Set aside.

2 For the cream, heat the vegetable oil in a saucepan over a medium heat and sauté the shallots and garlic until softened, but with no colour. Pour in the white wine and reduce by half, then pour in the fish stock and reduce that, too, by half. Add the cream and reduce to a creamy consistency. Pass through a sieve into a clean saucepan.

3 Preheat the oven to 200°C (180°C fan), Gas Mark 6.

4 Season the hake, place on a baking sheet lined with baking parchment and drizzle with a little rapeseed oil. Bake for 6–8 minutes, then remove from the oven and allow to rest for a few minutes.

5 Meanwhile, warm through the cream, finishing with the capers, cornichons and parsley and seasoning to taste with lemon juice, salt and pepper. Gently reheat the crushed potatoes.

6 Bring a saucepan of water to the boil and blanch the samphire for 5 seconds, then drain and dress with a little oil.

7 Serve the hake with the crushed potatoes, cream and samphire.

NUTRITIONAL INFO PER SERVING

ENERGY 369 KCAL | FAT 13.3G | CARBS 17.8G | (OF WHICH SUGARS) 3.6G | PROTEIN 26.2G

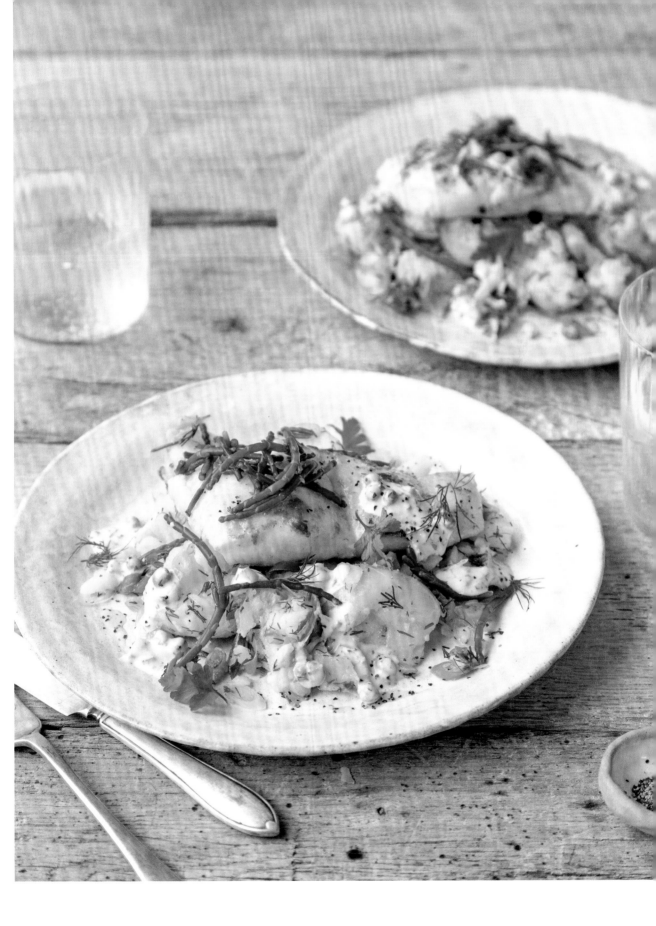

Grilled chicken, harissa-spiced chickpeas, dukkah

GLUTEN-FREE | DAIRY-FREE

SERVES 4

4 x 180–200g chicken
    breasts
2 teaspoons vegetable oil
½ small red onion (50g),
    finely chopped
2 garlic cloves, crushed or
    finely chopped
about ½ leek (50g),
    finely chopped
½ medium carrot (30g),
    finely chopped
½ teaspoon ground cumin
½ teaspoon ground
    turmeric
1 small red chilli, finely
    chopped
300g canned chickpeas,
    drained weight, rinsed
150ml chicken stock
    (gluten-free)
½ teaspoon cayenne pepper
1 teaspoon honey
1 teaspoon harissa paste
    (gluten-free)
15g flaked almonds
juice of 1½ lemons, plus
    lemon wedges to serve
5g coriander leaves,
    finely chopped

FOR THE DUKKAH
1 teaspoon coriander seeds
1 teaspoon cumin seeds
1 teaspoon cracked black
    peppercorns
1 teaspoon flaked almonds
sea salt (we use pink
    Himalayan) and freshly
    ground black pepper

1   Put everything for the dukkah in a dry frying pan and toast until fragrant and golden brown, then season, tip out into a bowl and set aside. Once cool, lightly crush the dukkah in a mortar and pestle.

2   Preheat the oven to 200°C (180°C fan), Gas Mark 6.

3   Season the chicken breasts and brush them all over with half the oil. Place a frying pan over a high heat. Sear the chicken, turning the breasts to get a lovely golden brown colour on all sides, then place in the oven for 12–14 minutes.

4   Meanwhile, heat the remaining oil in a heavy-based saucepan and sauté the onion, garlic, leek and carrot until softened but not coloured. Add the ground cumin, turmeric and chilli and cook slowly for a further 5 minutes. Add the chickpeas and chicken stock, season and allow to reduce by half.

5   Finish the chickpeas by adding the cayenne, honey, harissa paste, almonds, the juice of 1 lemon and most of the chopped coriander.

6   Once the chicken is cooked, allow to rest for a few minutes, then cut each breast into 3 pieces. Spoon the chickpeas into bowls, arrange the chicken breasts on top and crumble over the dukkah. Squeeze over the juice of the remaining half lemon and scatter with the remaining chopped coriander. Serve with lemon wedges on the side.

NUTRITIONAL INFO PER SERVING

ENERGY   378 KCAL | FAT   18.2G | CARBS   11.9G | (OF WHICH SUGARS) 9.5G | PROTEIN   44.2G

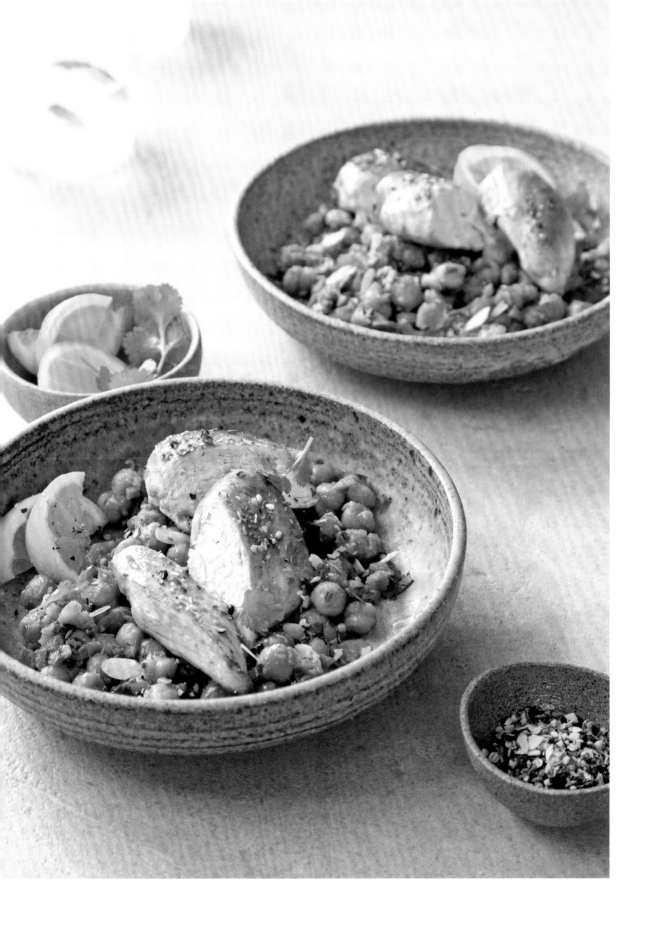

Coconut poached chicken leg, lentil dhal, crisp poppadoms

GLUTEN-FREE | DAIRY-FREE

SERVES 4

4 chicken legs

2 x 400ml cans of
   coconut milk

1 lemon grass stalk,
   finely chopped

5g root ginger, peeled and
   finely grated

5 garlic cloves, crushed or
   finely grated

5g chopped coriander stalks

4 plain poppadoms
   (gluten-free)

1 spring onion, finely
   chopped

FOR THE DHAL

1 tablespoon vegetable oil

2 garlic cloves, crushed or
   finely grated

2g root ginger, peeled and
   finely grated

½ small shallot, finely
   chopped

¼ teaspoon cumin seeds

½ teaspoon Madras curry
   powder (gluten-free)

½ teaspoon ground
   turmeric

50g red lentils, rinsed

200ml vegetable stock
   (gluten-free)

½ green chilli, deseeded and
   finely chopped

1 teaspoon finely chopped
   coriander leaves

juice of 1 lemon

sea salt (we use pink
   Himalayan) and freshly
   ground black pepper

1   Preheat the oven to 180°C (160°C fan), Gas Mark 4.

2   Score the skin of the chicken legs and place them in a deep baking tray. Add the coconut milk, lemon grass, ginger, garlic and chopped coriander stalks. Place in the oven for 1½ hours.

3   To make the dhal, heat the oil in a heavy-based saucepan and add the garlic, ginger and shallot. Cook for a few minutes until softened but not coloured. Add the cumin seeds and allow to cook for a further 5 minutes. Add the curry powder and turmeric and cook for a minute or so, until fragrant, then tip in the lentils and stock and allow to cook for 15–20 minutes until the lentils are soft but not overcooked. Finish with the green chilli, chopped coriander leaves and a little lemon juice and season well.

4   Meanwhile, remove the chicken legs from the cooking liquid and keep them hot. Pass the coconut milk mixture through a sieve into a saucepan and reduce it until it has a creamy consistency. Season to taste.

5   Cook the poppadoms according to the packet instructions, then break them into shards.

6   Place the dhal on plates or bowls and rest the chicken legs on top. Pour over the coconut sauce and scatter the dish with poppadom shards and the finely chopped spring onion.

NUTRITIONAL INFO PER SERVING

ENERGY 485 KCAL | FAT 31.8G | CARBS 24.2G | (OF WHICH SUGARS) 5.9G | PROTEIN 34.1G

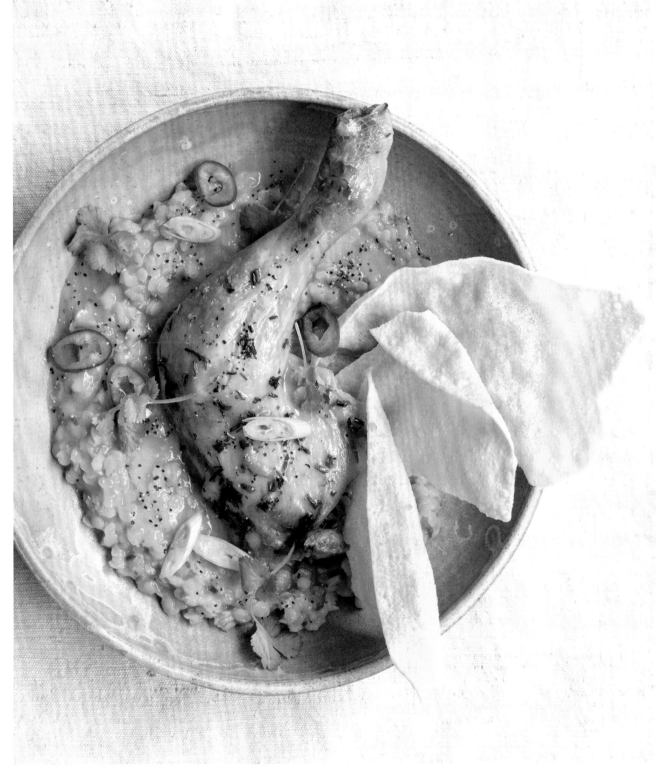

Chicken with sweet potato rosti and honey spiced vegetables

GLUTEN-FREE | DAIRY-FREE

SERVES 2

½ small red pepper (30g)
½ small yellow pepper (30g)
30g chunk of courgette
30g broccoli florets
½ medium carrot (30g)
½ small red onion (30g)
olive oil spray
2 medium chicken breasts
½ teaspoon garlic powder
(gluten-free)
sea salt (we use pink
Himalayan) and freshly
ground black pepper

FOR THE ROSTI

1 small sweet potato (125g),
well scrubbed
½ handful of mixed herb
leaves, such as basil,
coriander, thyme and
parsley, chopped, plus
more to serve
½ teaspoon cornflour
2 teaspoons olive oil
½ garlic clove, crushed
or finely grated
½ teaspoon freshly
grated nutmeg

FOR THE RAS EL
HANOUT HONEY
DRESSING

1 garlic clove, crushed or
finely grated
2 teaspoons olive oil
2 teaspoons honey
2 teaspoons harissa paste
(gluten-free)
½ teaspoon ras el hanout
(gluten-free)
2 teaspoons lemon juice
finely grated zest of
½ lemon, plus lemon
wedges to serve

1 Preheat the oven to 220°C (200°C fan), Gas Mark 7.

2 Chop the peppers, courgette, broccoli, carrot and red onion into even 1–2cm pieces. Put all the chopped vegetables on a baking sheet, spreading them out and not overcrowding them, season well, spray with olive oil spray and roast for around 25 minutes until tender, tossing once or twice during the roasting process.

3 Meanwhile, coarsely grate the unpeeled sweet potato on to a clean tea towel, then wrap it up and, over a sink, squeeze out as much moisture as possible. Tip into a mixing bowl and stir in all the other rosti ingredients, seasoning well.

4 Preheat a grill to medium.

5 Season the chicken with salt and pepper and the garlic powder. Mist a frying pan with olive oil spray, set it over a high heat and sear the chicken for 3–4 minutes, turning to get a good colour all over.

6 Place on a baking sheet and finish under the grill for 15–20 minutes, depending on thickness, or until cooked through but still moist.

NUTRITIONAL INFO PER SERVING

ENERGY 487 KCAL | FAT 21G | CARBS 30G | (OF WHICH SUGARS) 19G | PROTEIN 42G

7 Heat a frying pan. Divide the rosti mixture into 2 patties and cook for 5–6 minutes on each side until crisp, browned and cooked through.

8 Meanwhile, mix all the ingredients for the dressing well and blitz in a blender until emulsified.

9 Thickly slice the chicken on an angle and serve it on top of the sweet potato rosti, arrange the colourful vegetables around the edge, drizzle over some dressing and scatter with herbs. Serve the lemon wedges and the remaining dressing on the side.

Tip

Sweet potatoes are higher in fibre than some white potatoes. Beta-carotene – a beneficial phyto-chemical – gives sweet potatoes their bright orange colour.

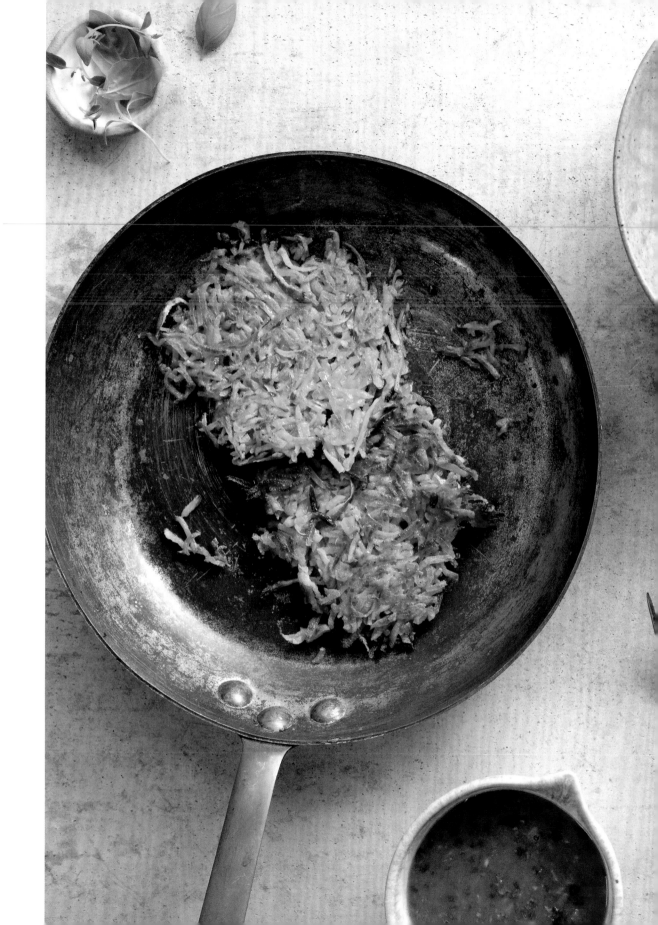

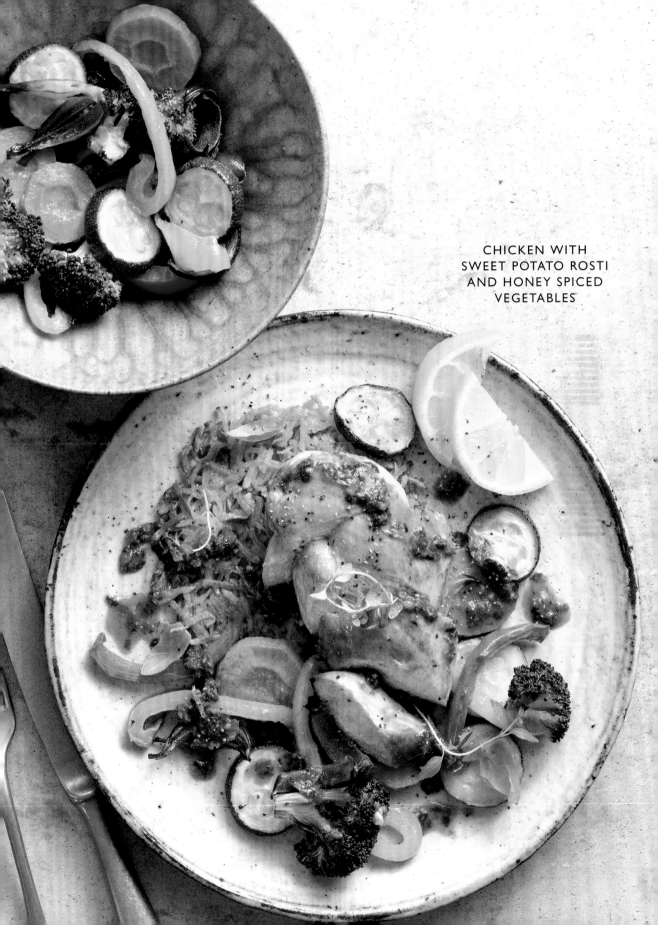

CHICKEN WITH
SWEET POTATO ROSTI
AND HONEY SPICED
VEGETABLES

Duck and bean burrito

with red cabbage and pomegranate slaw

SERVES 4

FOR THE BURRITO

2 teaspoons rapeseed oil

2 banana shallots, finely sliced

2 garlic cloves, crushed or finely chopped

5g root ginger, peeled and finely chopped

300g shredded hoisin duck (or see tip, below right)

100g canned kidney beans, drained weight, rinsed

20ml tamari

1 medium-small carrot (100g), julienned

100g chunk of mooli, julienned

50g coriander leaves

4 wholemeal tortilla wraps

olive oil spray

FOR THE SLAW

1 tablespoon grain mustard

2 tablespoons sherry vinegar

2 tablespoons rapeseed oil

100g chunk of red cabbage, shredded

1 medium-small carrot (100g), julienned

1 spring onion, finely sliced

25g cashew nuts, toasted and crushed

50g mint leaves, chopped

50g parsley leaves, chopped

50g pomegranate seeds

finely grated zest and juice of 1 lime

sea salt and freshly ground black pepper

1 To make the slaw, whisk the grain mustard, vinegar and oil together in a mixing bowl until well emulsified. Season well.

2 Toss in all the vegetables, nuts, herbs and fruit, season well and allow to marinate for 1 hour.

3 For the burritos, place a saucepan over a high heat with the oil, then add the shallots, garlic and ginger. Cook slowly until softened but not coloured. Add the shredded duck and kidney beans and allow to cook for a further 5 minutes, stirring frequently. Add the tamari, julienned vegetables and coriander, stir, then set aside and allow to cool.

4 Preheat the oven to 200°C (180°C fan), Gas Mark 6.

5 Evenly distribute the duck mixture in a thick line on the tortillas, fold the tortillas over each end of the line of filling, then roll away from you to form 4 burritos. Mist with olive oil spray, place in a roasting tin and cook for 12–15 minutes.

6 Remove the burritos from the oven, cut in half on an angle and serve with the slaw.

——— *Tip* ———

At Champneys, we aim to cater for all dietary needs. This delicious burrito can easily be adapted for a vegan diet by switching the duck for a plant-based pulled meat substitute.

NUTRITIONAL INFO PER SERVING

ENERGY 680 KCAL | FAT 31.7G | CARBS 46.8G | (OF WHICH SUGARS) 13.5G | PROTEIN 29.4G

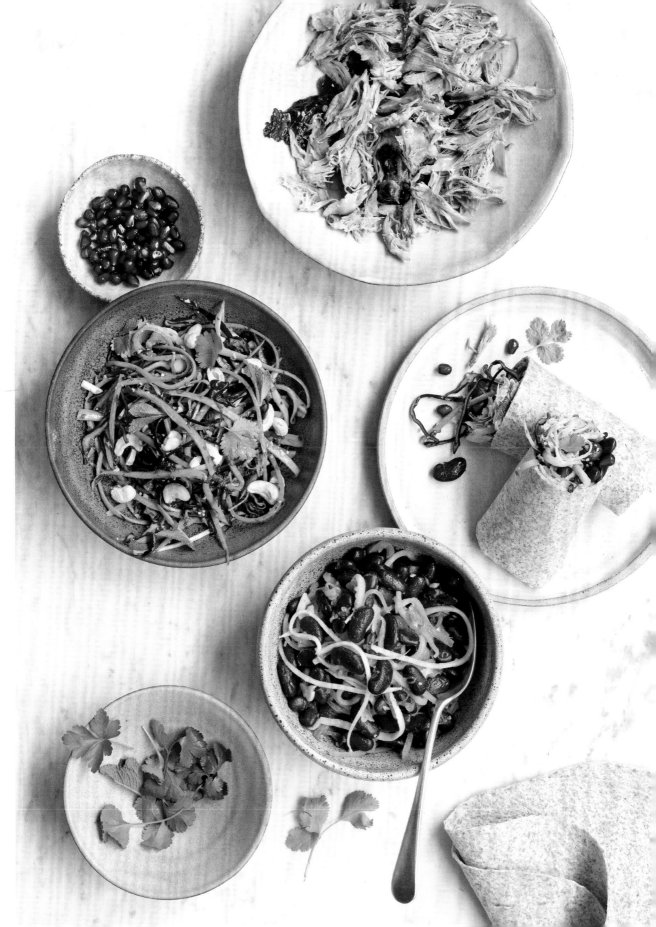

Grilled lamb cutlets, quinoa salad, tzatziki

GLUTEN-FREE

SERVES 4

FOR THE LAMB AND
MARINADE
2 tablespoons honey
50ml vegetable oil
4 garlic cloves, crushed or
    finely grated
1 teaspoon chilli powder
juice of 2 lemons
1 tablespoon pomegranate
    molasses
12 lamb cutlets
sea salt (we use pink
    Himalayan) and freshly
    ground black pepper
pomegranate seeds,
    to serve

FOR THE QUINOA
500g cooked quinoa
10g parsley leaves, finely
    chopped
5g mint leaves, shredded
about 2 plum tomatoes
    (200g), finely chopped
½ cucumber (200g),
    deseeded and
    finely chopped

1 garlic clove, crushed or
    finely grated
finely grated zest and juice
    of 1 lemon
50ml cold-pressed
    rapeseed oil

FOR THE TZATZIKI
250ml Greek yoghurt
¼ cucumber (100g),
    deseeded and
    finely chopped
5g mint leaves,
    finely chopped
5g coriander leaves,
    finely chopped
1 garlic clove, crushed or
    finely grated

1   The night before you want the lamb, whisk together all the ingredients for the marinade and season to taste. Place the lamb cutlets in a shallow tray and pour over the marinade, cover and refrigerate for 24 hours.

2   The next day, for the salad, place the quinoa, parsley, mint, tomatoes and cucumber in a bowl. Whisk together the garlic, lemon zest, juice and oil and stir into the quinoa mix, then season well.

3   Mix all the ingredients for the tzatziki together and season with a pinch of salt.

4   Remove the lamb cutlets from the marinade while you heat a griddle or frying pan over a very high heat until smoking hot. Cook the cutlets for 2 minutes on each side for medium-rare. Set the lamb aside to rest for 5 minutes.

5   Place the quinoa on plates, top with the lamb cutlets, spoon around the tzatziki and sprinkle with pomegranate seeds to serve.

NUTRITIONAL INFO PER SERVING

ENERGY 630 KCAL | FAT 36.9G | CARBS 50.4G | (OF WHICH SUGARS) 27.2G | PROTEIN 27.1G

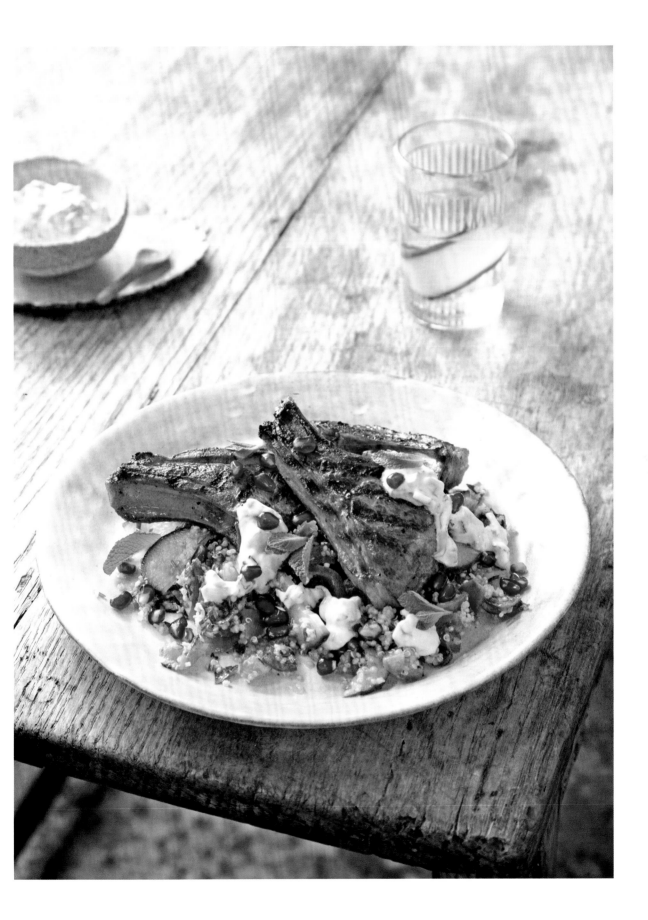

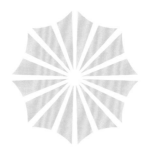

Desserts & Sweet Treats

Nutritious delicious bliss balls

VEGAN | GLUTEN-FREE | DAIRY-FREE

MAKES 8

200g oats (gluten-free)
20g sultanas
20g dried apricots, chopped
20g dried cranberries
20g pitted dates, chopped
20g pumpkin seeds
20g sunflower seeds
1 teaspoon mixed spice
30g hazelnut butter
80ml unsweetened rice milk
40–50g desiccated coconut,
    to coat

1   Place the oats, dried fruit and seeds and mixed spice in a bowl and stir to combine, or blend in a food processor for a smoother texture, if you prefer.

2   In a separate bowl, soften the nut butter in a microwave for around 20 seconds, then stir in the rice milk to make a smooth paste. Gradually add to the dried ingredients, mixing well until it forms a dough.

3   Use your hands to squeeze and shape the dough into 8 balls, around 50g each. Place the coconut on a plate.

4   Roll each ball in coconut and place on a freezerproof plate or baking sheet lined with baking parchment. Leave to firm up in the freezer for 30 minutes, or refrigerate for at least 2 hours, before serving.

5   Serve. Store any spares in a covered container in the fridge for up to 5 days.

Tip

To make these completely allergen-free, use pumpkin seed butter instead of nut butter and look for a brand of dried fruit that is free from sulphites.

NUTRITIONAL INFO PER BALL

ENERGY 204 KCAL | FAT 8.8G | CARBS 23G | (OF WHICH SUGARS) 6.1G | PROTEIN 5.9G

Black Forest bliss balls

VEGAN | GLUTEN-FREE | DAIRY-FREE

MAKES 8

75g cashew nuts
60g frozen cherries, thawed
8 large, soft pitted dates
2 tablespoons cacao nibs
1 heaped tablespoon raw
    cacao powder
25g desiccated coconut
1 tablespoon coconut oil
½ teaspoon vanilla extract
pinch of sea salt
small pinch of chilli powder

1 Put the cashews and half the cherries in a high-powered food processor and pulse to finely chop. Add the dates, cacao nibs and powder, the desiccated coconut, melted coconut oil, vanilla, salt and chilli. Pulse until the mixture is forming a dough.

2 Chop the remaining cherries and mix in by hand.

3 Use your hands to shape into 8 balls, around 50g each, and place on a freezerproof plate or baking sheet lined with baking parchment.

4 Leave to firm up in the freezer for 30 minutes, or refrigerate for at least 2 hours, before serving.

5 Serve. Store any spares in a covered container in the fridge for up to 5 days.

NUTRITIONAL INFO PER BALL

ENERGY 221 KCAL | FAT 17G | CARBS 12G | (OF WHICH SUGARS) 9.1G | PROTEIN 4.1G

Raspberry and lemon cheesecake bliss balls

VEGETARIAN | GLUTEN-FREE

MAKES 8

100g full-fat cream cheese
finely grated zest of
    1 lemon
3 tablespoons lemon juice
2 tablespoons xylitol
100g desiccated coconut
100g frozen raspberries,
    defrosted and drained

1 Place the cream cheese, lemon zest and juice and xylitol in a food processor, then blend until smooth and well combined. Add the desiccated coconut and blend again.

2 Roughly chop the raspberries with a sharp knife and mix in by hand.

3 Use your hands to shape into 8 balls, around 50g each, and place on a freezerproof plate or baking sheet lined with baking parchment.

4 Leave to firm up in the freezer for 30 minutes, or refrigerate for at least 2 hours, before serving.

5 Serve. Store any spares in a covered container in the fridge for up to 5 days.

NUTRITIONAL INFO PER BALL

ENERGY 140 KCAL | FAT 12G | CARBS 3.3G | (OF WHICH SUGARS) 1.9G | PROTEIN 1.8G

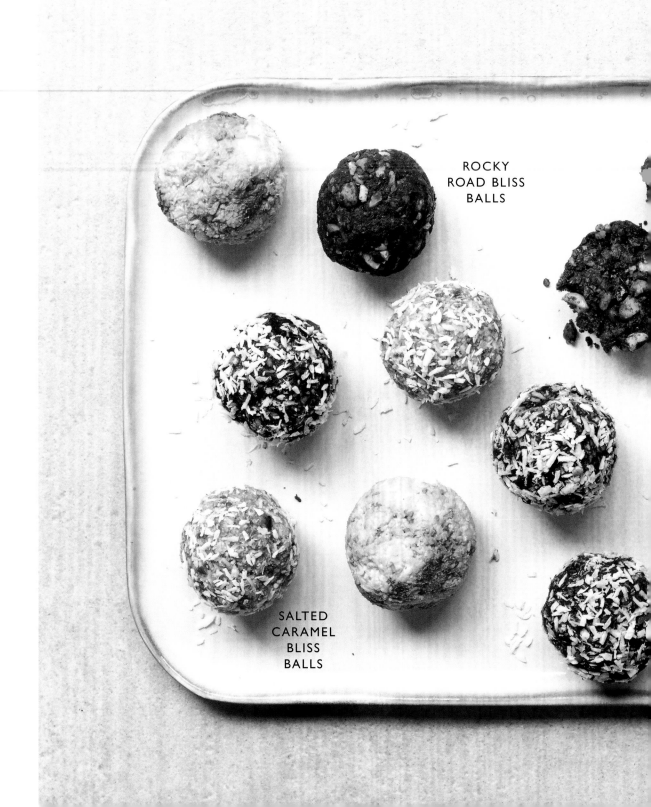

ROCKY
ROAD BLISS
BALLS

SALTED
CARAMEL
BLISS
BALLS

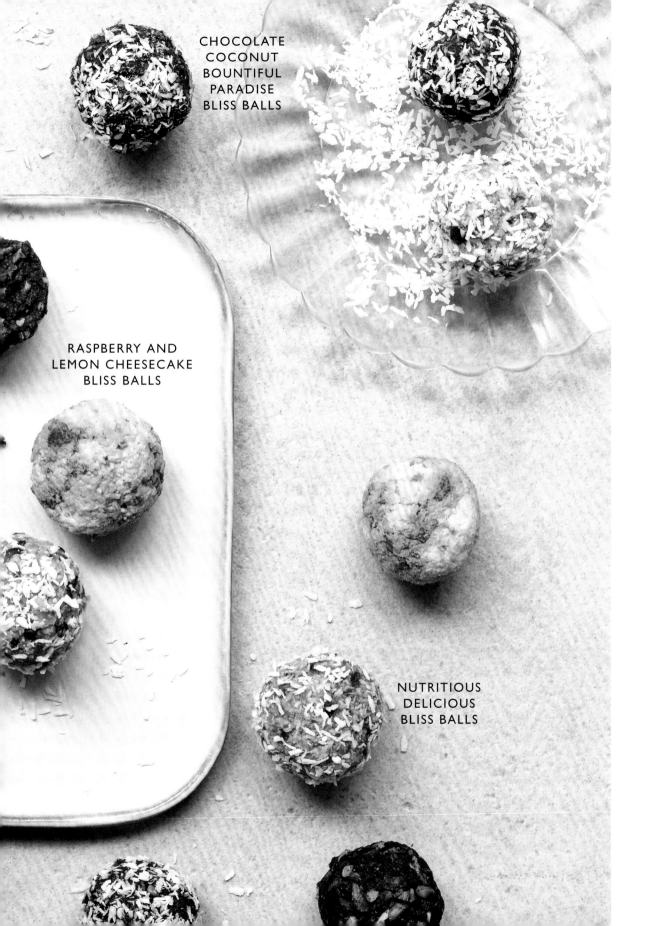

CHOCOLATE
COCONUT
BOUNTIFUL
PARADISE
BLISS BALLS

RASPBERRY AND
LEMON CHEESECAKE
BLISS BALLS

NUTRITIOUS
DELICIOUS
BLISS BALLS

Salted caramel bliss balls

VEGAN | GLUTEN-FREE | DAIRY-FREE

MAKES 8

150g pitted dates
50g ground almonds
50g oats (gluten-free)
75g desiccated coconut,
    plus 40–50g to coat
1 teaspoon sea salt (we use
    pink Himalayan)
1 teaspoon vanilla extract

1 Put the dates in a bowl, cover with warm water and soak for 30 minutes. Drain, reserving the liquid.

2 Put the drained dates in a food processor with the ground almonds, oats, 75g of the coconut, the salt and vanilla extract. Blend until smooth.

3 Check that the mixture is sufficiently moist to be able to roll into 8 balls. If not, add a little of the date soaking liquid.

4 Roll each ball in coconut and place on a freezerproof plate or baking sheet lined with baking parchment. Leave to firm up in the freezer for 30 minutes, or refrigerate for at least 2 hours.

5 Serve. Store any spares in a covered container in the fridge for up to 5 days.

NUTRITIONAL INFO PER BALL

ENERGY 232 KCAL | FAT 14G | CARBS 19G | (OF WHICH SUGARS) 14G | PROTEIN 3.8G

Rocky road bliss balls

VEGAN | GLUTEN-FREE | DAIRY-FREE

MAKES 8

50g pistachio nuts
30g cashew nuts
160g walnut pieces
60g pitted dates, chopped
30g raw cacao powder
1 teaspoon vanilla extract
30g dried cranberries
30g goji berries

1 Place half the pistachios and cashews in a high-powered food processor and quickly pulse to roughly crush. Tip into a bowl and set aside.

2 Place the walnuts, dates, cacao and vanilla into the food processor and blend at high speed until the mixture resembles sticky crumbs.

3 Roughly chop the remaining nuts and mix with the cranberries and goji berries. Add to the blended pistachio-cashew mixture, stir in the walnut mixture and combine well with a wooden spoon.

4 Roll into 8 balls and place on a freezerproof plate or baking sheet lined with baking parchment. Leave to firm up in the freezer for 30 minutes, or refrigerate for at least 2 hours, before serving.

5 Serve. Store any spares in a covered container in the fridge for up to 5 days.

NUTRITIONAL INFO PER BALL

ENERGY 264 KCAL | FAT 20G | CARBS 12G | (OF WHICH SUGARS) 9.3G | PROTEIN 7G

Chocolate coconut bountiful paradise bliss balls

VEGAN | GLUTEN-FREE | DAIRY-FREE

MAKES 8

100g raisins

50g oats (gluten-free)

50g sunflower seeds

50g pitted dates, chopped

50g raw cacao powder

30g desiccated coconut,
plus 40–50g to coat

1 tablespoon coconut oil,
melted (we use raw
organic extra-virgin)

1 Place all the ingredients, except the coconut for coating, into a high-powered food processor. Blend at high speed until the mixture resembles sticky crumbs.

2 Use your hands to shape into 8 balls. Place the 40–50g coconut on a plate.

3 Roll each ball in coconut and place on a freezerproof plate or baking sheet lined with baking parchment. Leave to firm up in the freezer for 30 minutes, or refrigerate for at least 2 hours, before serving.

4 Serve. Store any spares in a covered container in the fridge for up to 5 days.

Tip

Bliss balls are typically high in natural sugars as they're often packed with dried fruit. So, if you prefer a low-refined sugar option, these are the perfect tasty treat.

NUTRITIONAL INFO PER BALL

ENERGY 220 KCAL | FAT 12.2G | CARBS 21.1G | (OF WHICH SUGARS) 14.4G | PROTEIN 5.0G

Watermelon
berry pizza

VEGAN | GLUTEN-FREE | DAIRY-FREE

SERVES 4

200–250g dairy-free
    coconut yoghurt
    (gluten-free)
2.5cm-thick watermelon
    slice, taken from the
    widest part of a large
    watermelon
4 tablespoons desiccated
    coconut
2 tablespoons shredded
    mint leaves
8 large strawberries, sliced
large handful of blueberries
large handful of blackberries,
    halved
large handful of raspberries,
    halved
2 tablespoons flaked
    almonds, toasted

1 Spread the coconut yoghurt over the watermelon slice, using as much as you need for the size of your chosen slice, leaving a rim around the rind for people to hold their slices.

2 Sprinkle the watermelon pizza with coconut, mint leaves and the mixed berries, then top with the toasted flaked almonds.

3 Cut evenly into 8 pieces, as you would a pizza.

4 Serve in the middle of the table, so everyone can help themselves.

NUTRITIONAL INFO PER SERVING

ENERGY 129 KCAL | FAT 6.7G | CARBS 12G | (OF WHICH SUGARS) 9.6G | PROTEIN 2.0G

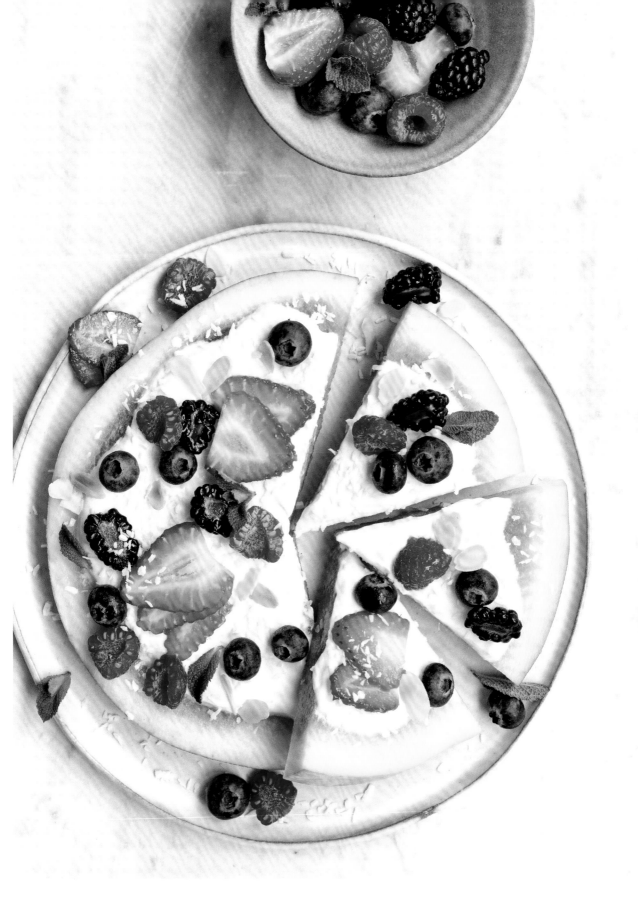

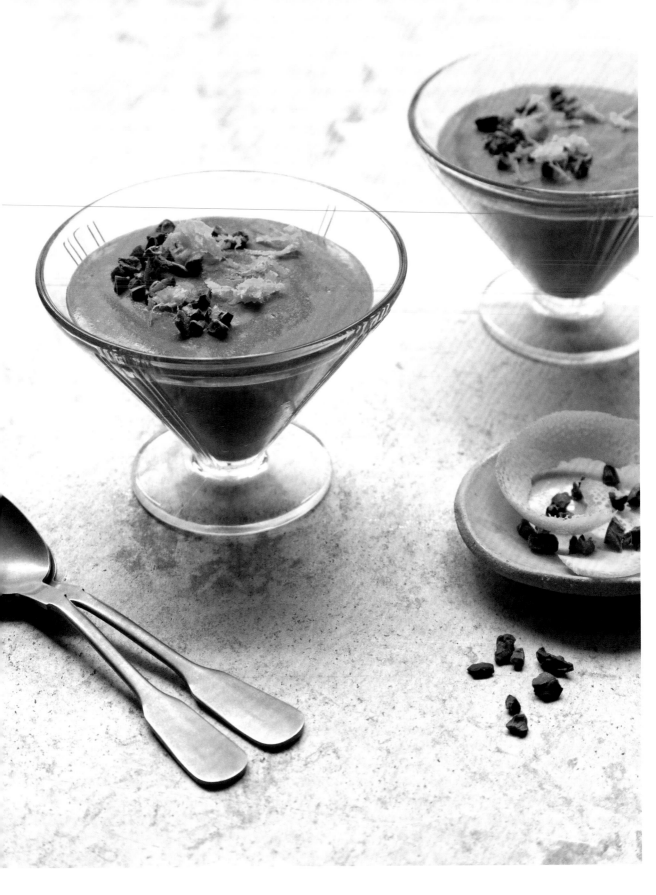

Dark chocolate
and orange mousse

VEGAN | GLUTEN-FREE | DAIRY-FREE

SERVES 2

50ml aquafaba (the
    liquid drained from
    canned chickpeas)
25g coconut sugar
¼ teaspoon cream
    of tartar
50g vegan dark chocolate, at
    least 70 per cent cocoa
    solids (gluten-free),
    chopped
50g silken tofu
10g cocoa powder, or
    raw cacao powder
finely grated zest and juice
    of 1 orange, plus orange
    zest to serve
10g cacao nibs (optional)

1 Whisk the aquafaba in a bowl with an electric
whisk, or using a stand mixer, until stiff. Gradually add
the coconut sugar and cream of tartar and continue
whisking for up to 10 minutes, until glossy and thick.

2 Put the chocolate in a heatproof bowl and set over
a saucepan of simmering water, making sure the bowl
does not touch the water. When the chocolate has
completely melted, remove the bowl from the saucepan
and leave to cool slightly. Using a hand blender, blend
the chocolate with the tofu and cocoa or cacao, a
squeeze of orange juice and the orange zest.

3 When the chocolate mix is cold, fold the aquafaba
whip into the chocolate mixture. Do NOT try to do this
the other way round – folding the chocolate into the
aquafaba – or it may split.

4 Divide the mousse between glasses, cover and place
in the fridge for a few hours.

5 Decorate with cacao nibs, if you like, and finely
grated orange zest.

NUTRITIONAL INFO PER SERVING

ENERGY 227 KCAL | FAT 12.7G | CARBS 26.1G | (OF WHICH SUGARS) 24.4G | PROTEIN 3.7 G

Blueberry and lemon eton mess

VEGETARIAN | GLUTEN-FREE

SERVES 2

100g frozen blueberries, defrosted, reserving the juices

finely grated zest and juice of 1 lemon

10g maple syrup

150g natural yoghurt

150g plant-based whipping cream (gluten-free)

½ teaspoon vanilla extract

2 teaspoons lemon curd

80g fresh blueberries

1 ready-made meringue nest, crushed

10g flaked almonds

1   In a bowl, mix the juice that came out of the defrosted blueberries with the lemon juice, half the lemon zest and the maple syrup.

2   Put the yoghurt in a separate bowl with the plant-based cream, vanilla and lemon curd. Using an electric whisk, beat until light and airy.

3   Divide the blueberry-maple mix between 2 glasses and scatter with the defrosted blueberries. Top with half the yoghurt mix, then a layer of half the fresh blueberries and half the crushed meringue. Now spoon over the rest of the yoghurt, crumble on the last of the meringue and scatter with a few of the remaining fresh blueberries.

4   Sprinkle with the flaked almonds, remaining fresh blueberries and lemon zest and serve.

NUTRITIONAL INFO PER SERVING

ENERGY 385 KCAL | FAT 18.9G | CARBS 25.2G | (OF WHICH SUGARS) 23.4G | PROTEIN 7.1G

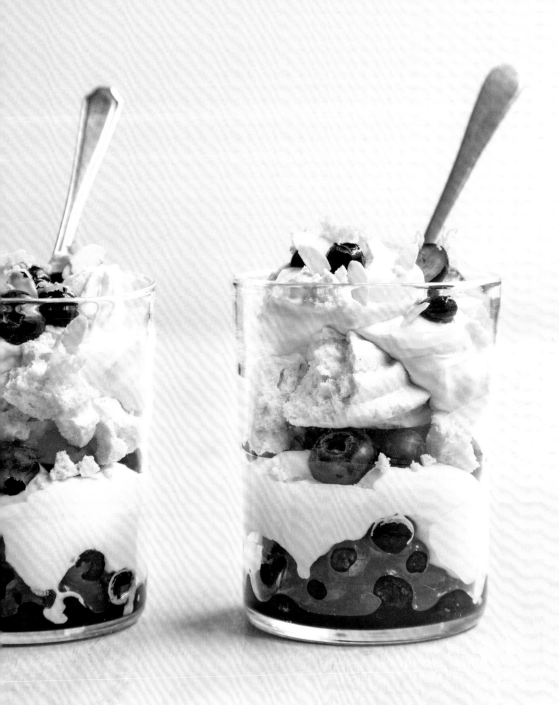

White chocolate macadamia blondie

with blueberry compote

VEGAN | GLUTEN-FREE | DAIRY-FREE

MAKES 4

1 teaspoon coconut oil
(we use raw organic
extra-virgin)
180g cashew butter
360g canned chickpeas,
drained weight, rinsed
105g maple syrup
90g xylitol
3 tablespoons unsweetened
almond milk
3 teaspoons vanilla extract
¾ teaspoon baking powder
1½ teaspoons bicarbonate
of soda
pinch of sea salt
105g vegan white chocolate
(gluten-free), chopped
60g macadamia nuts,
chopped
plant-based cream (gluten-
free), to serve (optional)

FOR THE COMPOTE
240g frozen blueberries,
defrosted (juices
reserved)
3 tablespoons lemon juice
1½ teaspoons vanilla
extract
3 tablespoons xylitol
(optional)

1 Before starting to make the blondies, ensure all the ingredients are at room temperature, for better blending.

2 Preheat the oven to 200°C (180°C fan), Gas Mark 6. Oil a 20cm square baking tin with the coconut oil.

3 Melt the cashew butter a little in the microwave, then put it in the bowl of a high-powered blender. Add the chickpeas, maple syrup, xylitol, almond milk, vanilla extract, baking powder, bicarbonate of soda and salt. Blend until creamy and smooth (2–5 minutes, depending on your blender).

4 Once the blondie mix is smooth, add half the white chocolate and mix by hand to combine well. Mix in half the macadamias, pour into the prepared tin and spread out evenly. Sprinkle the remaining white chocolate and nuts over the top.

5 Bake in the preheated oven for 20–25 minutes until the edges just pull away from the tin and the top is set and slightly golden brown. Don't overcook, as you want the blondies to remain fudgey in the centre. Let cool for at least 15 minutes to firm up before slicing.

6 Meanwhile, for the blueberry compote, combine the blueberries with the lemon juice and vanilla extract in a small saucepan. Heat until the compote reduces and becomes sticky. Taste and see if you want to sweeten the compote with the xylitol (remember you will be serving it with the sweet blondies).

7 Serve the blondies with the compote and plant-based cream, if you like.

NUTRITIONAL INFO PER SERVING

ENERGY 313 KCAL | FAT 19G | CARBS 29G | (OF WHICH SUGARS) 10G | PROTEIN 6.1G

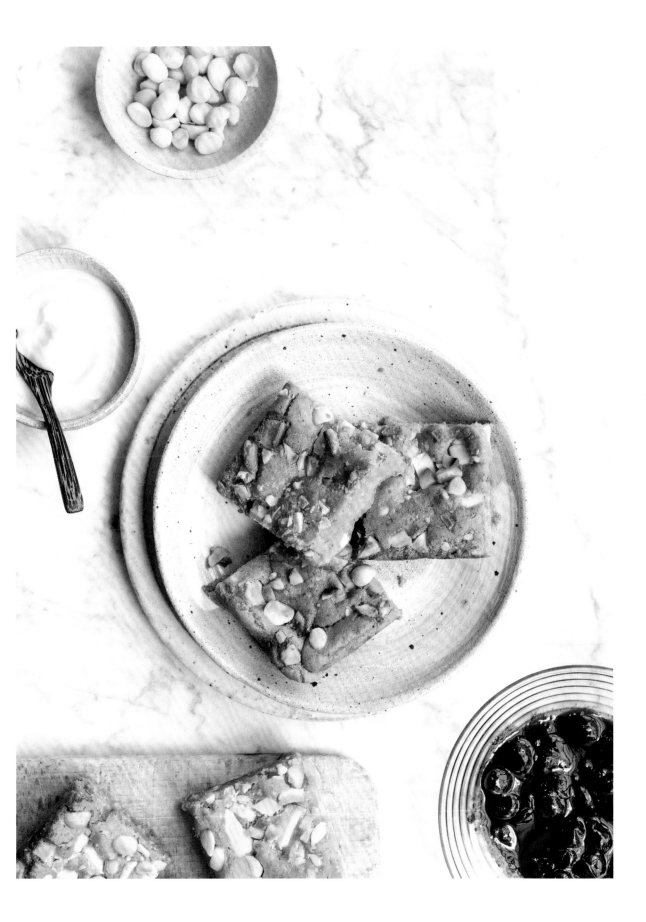

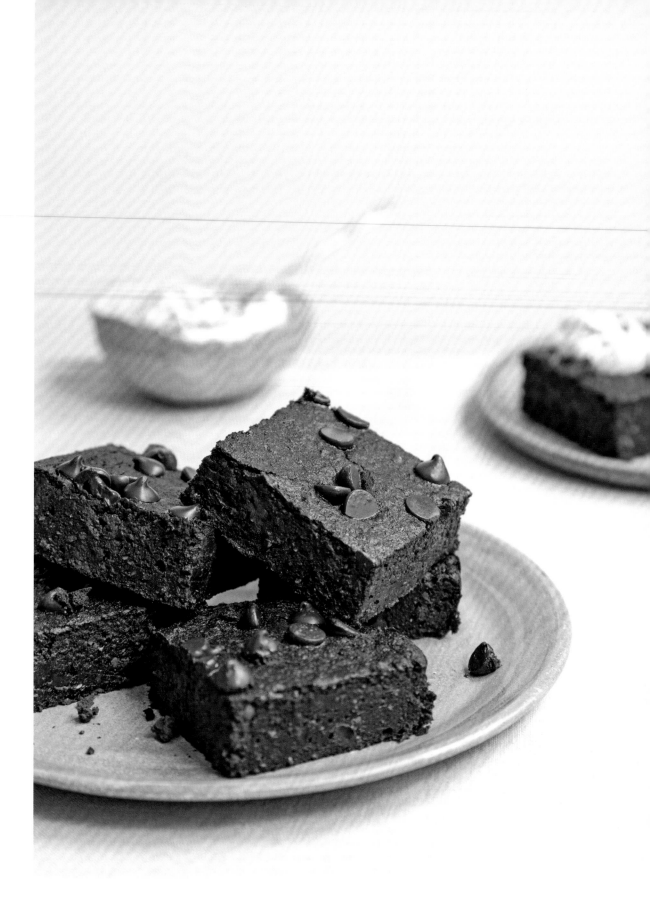

Beetroot chocolate brownie

VEGAN | GLUTEN-FREE | DAIRY-FREE

MAKES 4 AS DESSERT OR 8 AS A SNACK

50g ground flaxseed

125ml water

40g coconut oil, plus more for the tin (we use raw organic extra-virgin)

300g cooked natural (not pickled) beetroot

50g coconut sugar

150ml oat milk (gluten-free)

1 teaspoon vanilla extract

100g buckwheat flour

50g cocoa powder, or raw cacao powder

½ teaspoon baking powder (gluten-free)

100g vegan dark chocolate chips (gluten-free)

pinch of sea salt

plant-based cream (gluten-free), to serve

1 Combine the flaxseed in a bowl with the measured water and leave to thicken for 5 minutes.

2 Preheat the oven to 200°C (180°C fan), Gas Mark 6 and oil a 20cm square baking tin with coconut oil.

3 Roughly chop and blend the beetroot in a high-powered blender until completely smooth.

4 Melt the coconut oil in a small saucepan, then pour it into a mixing bowl and stir in the coconut sugar. Add the flax mix, the oat milk, vanilla extract and beetroot purée.

5 Sift in the buckwheat flour, cocoa or cacao powder and baking powder and gently fold the mixture together.

6 Add half the chocolate chips with a pinch of salt and gently fold them in.

7 Pour half the mixture into the prepared tin, sprinkle half the remaining chocolate chips on top, then pour over the rest of the brownie mixture and scatter on the remaining chocolate chips. Smooth the surface with a spatula. Bake for 25–30 minutes until the edges are crisp and set but the centre is a still a little fudgey.

8 Leave to cool in the baking tin for at least 15 minutes.

9 Turn out and leave the brownies to cool to room temperature before cutting into 4 or 8 and serving, with some plant-based cream, if you like.

NUTRITIONAL INFO PER SERVING

ENERGY 258 KCAL | FAT 13.7G | CARBS 29.6G | (OF WHICH SUGARS) 18.8G | PROTEIN 5.8G

Labneh, roast apple,
salted caramel almond drizzle

VEGETARIAN | GLUTEN-FREE

SERVES 2

2 large eating apples
½ teaspoon ground
   cinnamon
1 teaspoon xylitol
olive oil spray
200g labneh, or very
   good-quality, very thick
   Greek yoghurt
1 teaspoon maple syrup
½ teaspoon vanilla extract
10g almond butter
2 tablespoons caramel syrup
   (gluten-free)
50ml soya yoghurt
   (gluten-free)
10g flaked almonds
sea salt (we use pink
   Himalayan)

1 Preheat the oven to 200°C (180°C fan), Gas Mark 6.

2 Cut the apples into wedges, some peeled, some with skin on. Sprinkle them with the cinnamon and xylitol and mist with olive oil spray. Place them on a baking sheet lined with baking parchment and roast in the oven for 10–15 minutes until softened and browned to your liking. Leave to cool.

3 In a mixing bowl, combine the labneh or very thick yoghurt with the maple syrup, vanilla and a pinch of salt. Set aside.

4 In another bowl, combine the almond butter, caramel syrup, soya yoghurt and another pinch of salt. Using an electric whisk, beat until well aerated.

5 Divide the yoghurt mixture between bowls, top it with the roast apple wedges and drizzle over the salted caramel sauce. Scatter with flaked almonds and serve.

Tip

If you have a local Middle Eastern, Greek or Turkish shop, they usually sell tubs of labneh near the yoghurt.

NUTRITIONAL INFO PER SERVING

ENERGY 227 KCAL | FAT 10.7G | CARBS 22.6G | (OF WHICH SUGARS) 21.3G | PROTEIN 6.7G

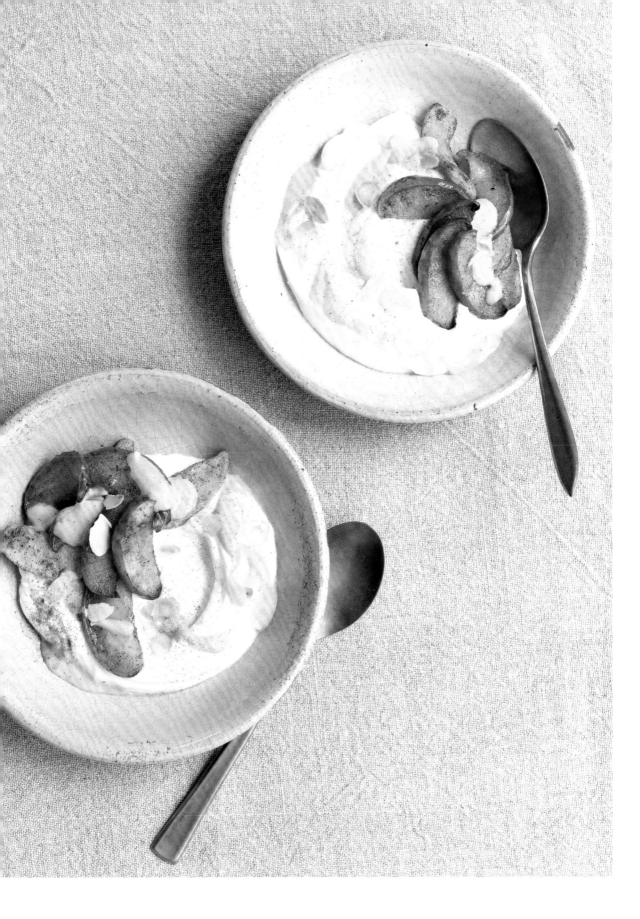

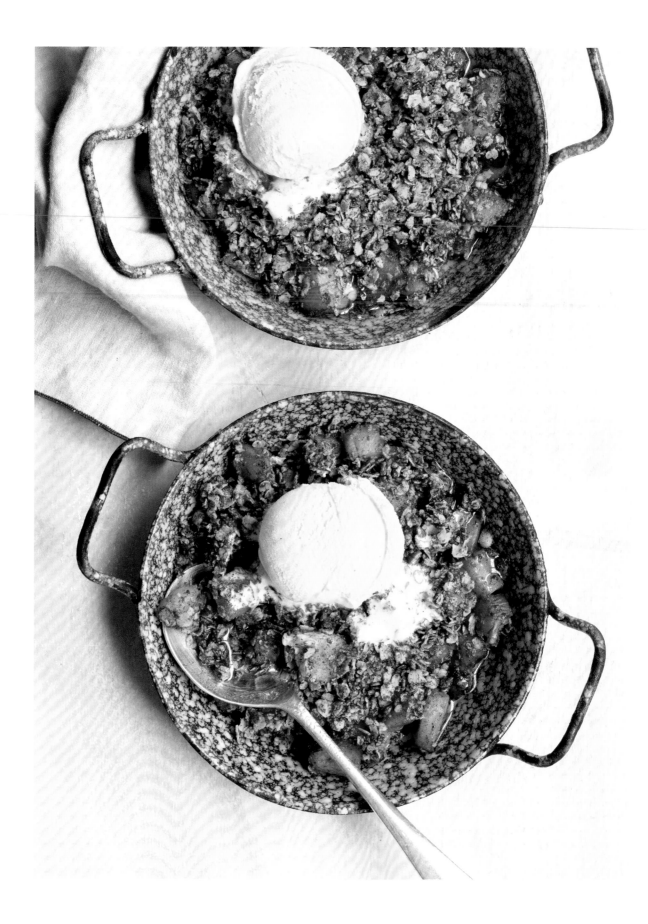

Butternut apple crumble

VEGAN | GLUTEN-FREE | DAIRY-FREE

SERVES 4

FOR THE CRUMBLE
50g oats (gluten-free)
20g coconut oil, melted
   (we use raw organic
   extra-virgin)
¼ teaspoon sea salt (we
   use pink Himalayan)
2 teaspoons ground
   cinnamon
1 teaspoon freshly
   ground nutmeg
½ teaspoon ground ginger

FOR THE FILLING
75g butternut squash,
   peeled weight, cut into
   1cm chunks
about 2 eating apples (250g),
   peeled, cored and cut into
   1cm chunks
1 teaspoon ground
   cinnamon
1 teaspoon arrowroot
   powder (gluten-free)
1 teaspoon cornflour
10g maple syrup
1 tablespoon xylitol

1   Preheat the oven to 200°C (180°C fan), Gas Mark 6.

2   In a mixing bowl, combine all the ingredients for the crumble. If making this ahead of time, cover and refrigerate until needed.

3   Combine all the ingredients for the filling and divide it between 4 ovenproof dishes, then top with the crumble.

4   Bake for 25–30 minutes, or until the filling is bubbling and the crumble is golden brown.

5   Allow to cool for 5–10 minutes before serving.

_____ *Tip* _____

Try serving this delicious dessert with your favourite cream, ice cream or custard. Whipped coconut cream mixed with a little maple syrup and vanilla extract is divine, and keeps the dish plant-based and dairy-free.

NUTRITIONAL INFO PER SERVING

ENERGY 230 KCAL | FAT 7.7G | CARBS 36G | (OF WHICH SUGARS) 16G | PROTEIN 4.5G

Rhubarb, ginger and custard

VEGAN | GLUTEN-FREE | DAIRY-FREE

SERVES 2

150g fresh rhubarb
finely grated zest and juice
    of ½ orange
2 teaspoons maple syrup
½ teaspoon peeled and
    finely grated root ginger
2 tablespoons water
100g frozen and defrosted
    rhubarb, or canned
    rhubarb, drained
1 teaspoon finely chopped
    stem ginger
150g dairy-free custard
    (gluten-free)
1 ginger nut biscuit
    (gluten-free), crushed

1   Trim and cut the fresh rhubarb into 2.5cm pieces. Place it in a pan with the orange zest and juice, half the maple syrup, the root ginger and measured water.

2   Set over a medium heat and bring to the boil, then reduce the heat to a simmer and cook gently for 6–8 minutes, until the rhubarb is cooked but still holds its shape. Set aside to cool to room temperature.

3   In the bowl of a food processor, or a bowl you can use with a hand blender, mix the defrosted or canned and drained rhubarb, the remaining maple syrup and half the stem ginger. Blend until smooth.

4   Heat the dairy-free custard until slightly warm.

5   Arrange pieces of the cooled poached rhubarb, the rhubarb purée, slightly warm custard and crushed ginger nut biscuit in 2 bowls, scatter with the remaining stem ginger, then serve straight away.

NUTRITIONAL INFO PER SERVING

ENERGY 135 KCAL | FAT 3.2G | CARBS 19.7G | (OF WHICH SUGARS) 9.8G | PROTEIN 3.7G

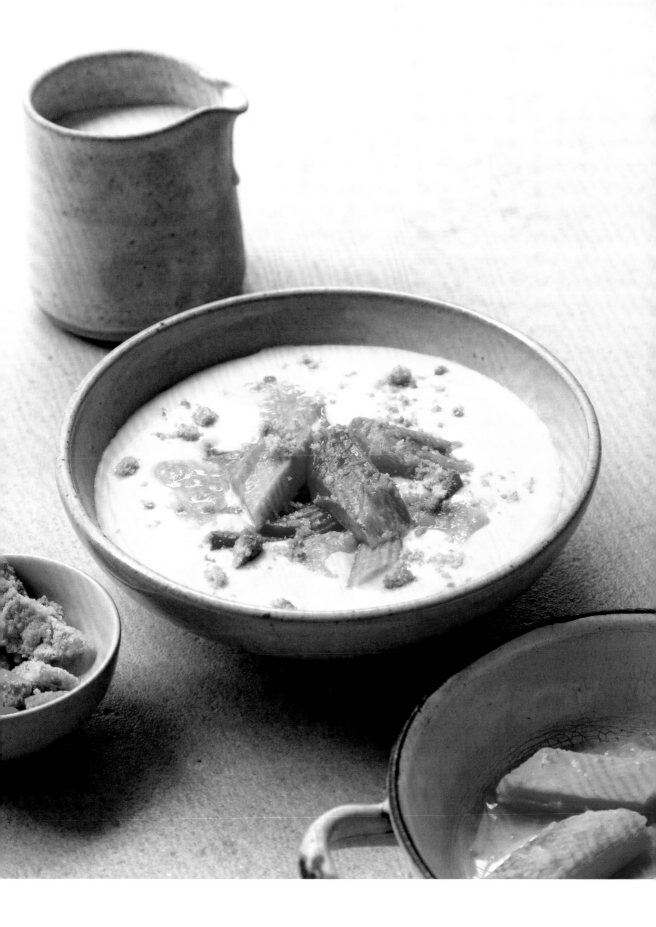

Lemon, poppy seed and courgette cake
with blackberry compote

SERVES 16

2 teaspoons olive oil
300g wholemeal self-raising
    flour
1 teaspoon baking powder
1 teaspoon ground
    cinnamon
pinch of sea salt (we use
    pink Himalayan)
4 large eggs
250g unsalted butter, or
    plant-based butter,
    softened
200g xylitol
1 teaspoon vanilla extract
2 large courgettes (400g),
    grated
finely grated zest and juice
    of 2 lemons, plus more
    zest (optional) to serve
6 tablespoons poppy seeds
natural yoghurt, to serve

FOR THE GLAZE
1½ tablespoons caster
    sugar
1 tablespoon lemon juice

FOR THE COMPOTE
300g frozen blackberries
100ml apple juice

1 Preheat the oven to 200°C (180°C fan), Gas Mark 6.

2 Use the oil to oil a loaf tin, then line the base with baking parchment.

3 Put the flour in a bowl and stir in the baking powder, cinnamon and a large pinch of salt.

4 In a separate bowl, beat together the eggs, butter, xylitol and vanilla extract. Mix the wet ingredients into the flour mixture until combined.

5 Coarsely grate the courgettes and squeeze out any excess liquid, using your hands or a muslin cloth.

6 Stir the courgettes, lemon zest and juice and poppy seeds into the batter. Pour into the prepared tin and bake for 60–75 minutes, or until a skewer inserted into the middle comes out clean. Leave in the tin to cool.

7 Mix the ingredients for the glaze, then pour it over the cake while still in the tin. Leave the glaze to set.

8 For the compote, place the fruit and juice in a saucepan over a medium heat. Once bubbling, reduce the heat slightly and use a wooden spoon to muddle and mash the fruit. Simmer for 3–4 minutes to reduce and thicken, then leave the compote to cool.

9 To serve, cut into slices and serve with the compote and yoghurt, sprinkling over lemon zest, if you like.

NUTRITIONAL INFO PER SERVING

ENERGY 304 KCAL | FAT 18G | CARBS 30.3G | (OF WHICH SUGARS) 21.2G | PROTEIN 9.3G

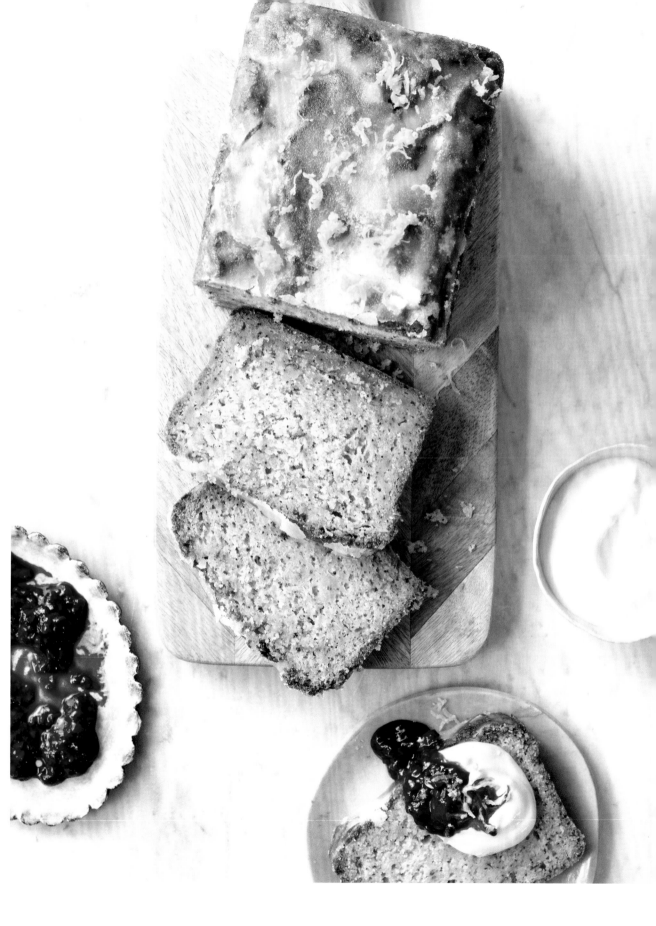

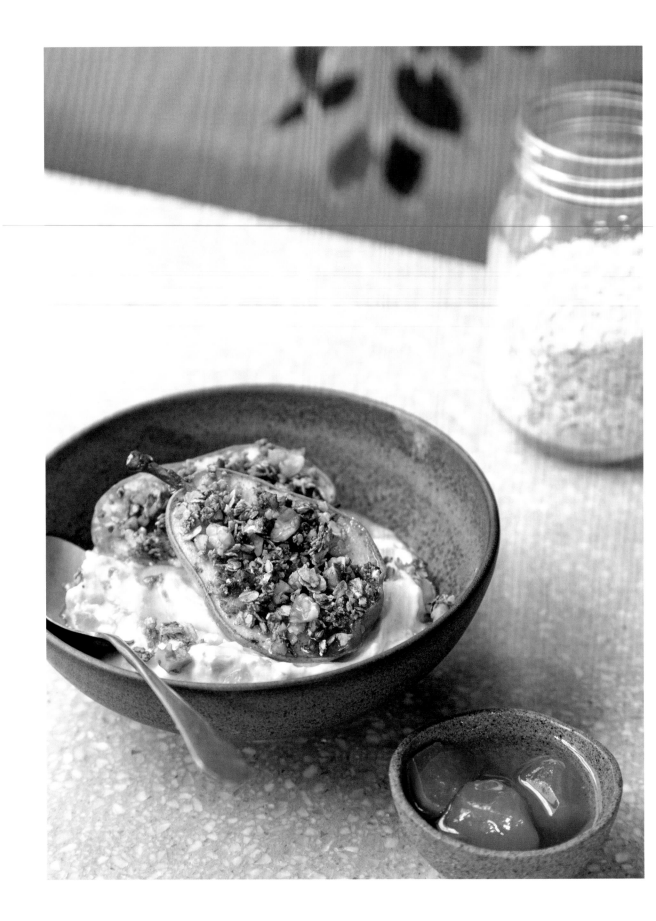

Roast pear, ginger cream, walnut crunch

VEGAN | GLUTEN-FREE | DAIRY-FREE

SERVES 2

2 medium pears
1 tablespoon maple syrup
1 teaspoon ground
   cinnamon
2 tablespoons oats
   (gluten-free)
2 tablespoons chopped
   walnuts
4 tablespoons plant-based
   cream (gluten-free)
1 teaspoon ground ginger
1 tablespoon finely chopped
   stem ginger

1 Preheat the oven to 200°C (180°C fan), Gas Mark 6.

2 Halve the pears, scoop out the cores and place on a baking sheet.

3 Brush the maple syrup over each pear and sprinkle with the cinnamon, oats and walnuts.

4 Bake in the oven for 30 minutes, then remove and allow to cool.

5 Whip the cream with the ground and stem ginger and serve with the pears with their crunchy cinnamon, oat and walnut coating.

NUTRITIONAL INFO PER SERVING

ENERGY 289 KCAL | FAT 6.1G | CARBS 25.4G | (OF WHICH SUGARS) 15.1G | PROTEIN 3.3G

Vegan tiramisu

VEGAN | GLUTEN-FREE | DAIRY-FREE

SERVES 6–8

FOR THE BASE

120ml unsweetened
    almond milk

80g xylitol

1 teaspoon vanilla extract

4 tablespoons Amaretto
    liqueur

4 large slices of white vegan
    bread (gluten-free)

4 teaspoons cocoa powder,
    or raw cacao powder

80g vegan dark chocolate,
    at least 70 per cent cocoa
    solids (gluten-free)

FOR THE MOCHA
CREAM TOPPING

150g unsalted cashews, or
    cashew pieces

400g extra-firm silken tofu,
    drained and pressed to
    remove excess water

6 tablespoons very strong
    brewed coffee, such
    as espresso

120g xylitol

2 teaspoons vanilla extract

1 For the topping, put the cashews in a bowl, cover with cold water and set in a cool place to soak for at least 4–6 hours, or up to 24 hours.

2 To make the base, put the almond milk and xylitol in a small saucepan and heat gently until the xylitol has dissolved. Add the vanilla extract and Amaretto, mix, then turn off the heat.

3 Remove and discard the crusts from the bread. Cut the bread into triangles and arrange it in a small dish. Pour the almond milk mixture evenly over the bread, sprinkle with half the cocoa powder, or raw cacao powder, and set aside.

4 To make the mocha cream, drain the cashews. Blitz the soaked cashews in a high-powered blender until smooth, then add the pressed silken tofu, coffee, xylitol and vanilla. Blitz the cream again until everything is very smooth and well integrated. Freeze for at least 6 hours, or overnight, to firm up.

5 Spoon the mocha cream evenly over the bread base, then sprinkle the rest of the cocoa over evenly.

6 Chill for at least 1 hour.

7 Evenly grate over the chocolate, then serve.

Tip

To ensure your tiramisu is fully vegan, make sure you choose a brand of gluten-free bread that doesn't contain egg, and a brand of dark chocolate that doesn't contain milk.

NUTRITIONAL INFO PER SERVING

ENERGY 353 KCAL | FAT 19G | CARBS 34G | (OF WHICH SUGARS) 6.5G | PROTEIN 14G

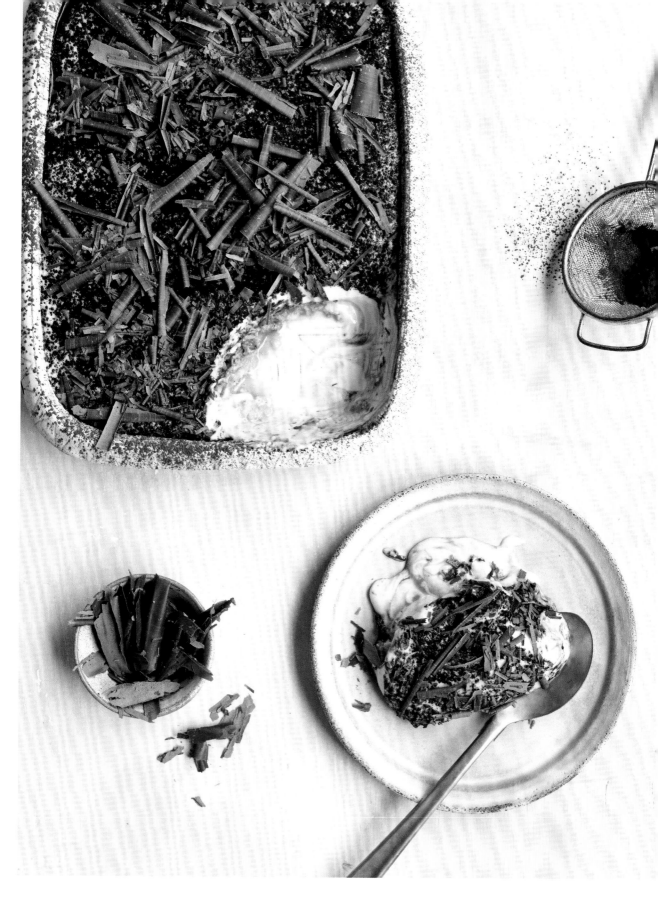

Index

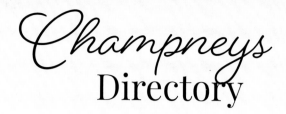

Champneys
Directory

Champneys have three types of spa location: spa resorts, spa hotels and city spas.

SPA RESORTS

A 'spa resort' is a countryside location packed with amenities centred on health and wellbeing. They combine gym and leisure facilities, massages and treatments, swimming pools, saunas and steam rooms among other activities. Champneys operate four of the most luxurious spa resorts in the UK. All are home to innovative and world-class treatments, cosy relaxation areas, show-stopping swimming pools, high-tech thermal experiences, nutritionist-approved menus and spa retreats to nourish you from the inside out.

Champneys Tring, in the rolling Hertfordshire hills, has been pioneering and perfecting health and wellbeing treatments since 1925. Close enough to London to be reachable, but far enough away to be peaceful, it's full of modern and traditional treatments, as well as the unique Marine and Wellness Spa.

Champneys Tring, Chesham Road, Tring HP23 6HY

Tucked away in the beautiful South Downs in Hampshire is **Champneys Forest Mere**, the perfect blend of spa resort and countryside hideaway. State-of-the-art facilities and a range of thermal spa treatments include an outdoor pool and warm, cosy spaces, far from the hustle and bustle of modern life.

Champneys Forest Mere, Portsmouth Road, Liphook GU30 7JG

Champneys Henlow, a gorgeous Georgian manor in Bedfordshire, is as close as most of us will ever get to living a *Downton Abbey* lifestyle. World-class spa facilities, 40 treatment rooms, 20 exercise classes a day and tennis and badminton courts means that there is something at this resort for everyone.

Champneys Henlow, Coach Road, Henlow SG16 6BT

Near Ashby-de-la-Zouch in the heart of the Midlands, **Champneys Springs** is the UK's first purpose-built health spa. It's the sportiest Champneys location and its pitches and training facilities are often used by professional athletes, but it's backed up with a plethora of pampering treatments and spaces to relax, too.

Champneys Springs, Gallow Lane, Ashby-de-la-Zouch DE12 7HD

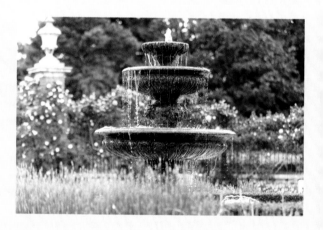

SPA HOTELS

A 'spa hotel' combines the luxurious facilities and treatments of a spa with top-quality accommodation and dining. They're perfect for overnight stays and weekends away, where you can feel spoiled and pampered by day and wined and dined by night. There are two Champneys luxury spa hotels. Both feature elegant interiors, gourmet dining, glamorous bars with extensive cocktail and wine lists, afternoon tea and a Champneys spa for that all-important relaxation.

Champneys Eastwell Manor is a picture-postcard spa hotel, ideal for a countryside break in the Garden of England. A break here gives you access to health and beauty treatments, indoor and outdoor heated swimming pools, gym, sauna, nature trails and top-class dining in the brasserie.

Eastwell Manor, Eastwell Park, Boughton Lees, Ashford TN25 4HR

Champneys Mottram Hall in Cheshire is a Grade II-listed building, set in 270 acres of landscaped gardens and equipped with £15 million of spa facilities and features. You'll also find an 18-hole championship golf course, a cutting-edge gym and a range of delicious food and drink options throughout the day.

Mottram Hall, Wilmslow Road, Mottram SK10 4QT

CITY SPAS

The Beauty House by Champneys
23 Market Place
St Albans
Hertfordshire
AL3 5DP

Champneys City Spa, Enfield
2 Hatton Walk
Palace Exchange
Enfield
EN2 6BP

Champneys City Spa, Milton Keynes
Boots, Crown Walk
centre:mk
Milton Keynes
Buckinghamshire
MK9 3AH

Acknowledgements

A thank you to all the team at Octopus Publishing Group who have made this book possible. Special mention to Lucy, Nicky, Sybella, Holly and Holly for all of their editorial, kitchen and creative input.

A special thank you to Dorothy Purdew OBE, who has been passionate about the Champneys food principles across the decades. Dorothy started her first business, Weight Guard, in 1970 and was one of the first to recommend a low-carbohydrate diet for people wanting to lose weight. Even today she can be found at chefs' food tastings, or talking to guests and wanting their feedback on a daily basis.

Finally, to all the Champneys chefs and kitchen teams. They are up with the lark to ensure that all our guests experience delicious food from dawn until dusk.

Special thanks to the Champneys Head Chefs: Andrew Green, Marius Ionut-Dan, Marc Petit, Hendrick Schirm, David Terrell and Matthew Underwood.